CONTENTS

Investigations

Subtle Abuse
in Adult Social Care

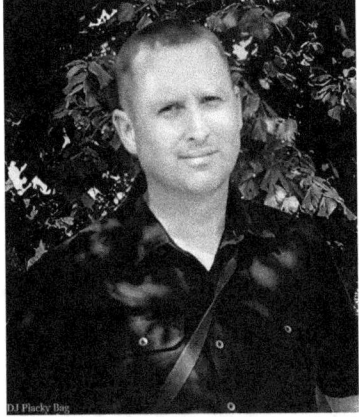

By Alexander Hylton Parker

Copyright © 2020 Alexander Hylton Parker
Visit Alex H Parker websites for more information and to get to know the author:
www.alexhparker.com
www.plackybag.co.uk
www.plesseycastle.com

Published by: Alex H Parker & Plessey Castle

Email: arccstic@gmail.com
Website: www.alexhparker.com

Any resemblance to real persons or other real-life entities is purely coincidental. All characters and other entities appearing in this work are fictitious examples unless otherwise stated. Any resemblance to real persons, dead or alive, or other real-life entities, past or present, is purely coincidental, with the exception of Santa Clause, who is real. I have photos.

PREFACE

As the author of this book, I feel it is important to acknowledge that it is a departure from my previous works. This book is not lighthearted or humorous, but rather it tackles some difficult and unsettling subjects that may be challenging for some readers to digest. It focuses on an important issue within the social care system, but it is an issue that many people would prefer to avoid or ignore.

As the book progresses, readers will be taken on a journey into the mind of the abuser, a place that angels would fear to tread. The book explores the values and traits commonly exhibited by abusive individuals, shedding light on the motivations and behaviors that underpin abuse. By confronting this uncomfortable and unsettling subject matter, the book provides valuable insights into the psychology of abuse and the individuals who perpetrate it. The exploration of the abuser's mindset is a crucial part of understanding and addressing abuse within the social care system. By gaining a deeper understanding of the motivations and behaviors of abusive individuals, social care workers and organizations can better recognize warning signs and take proactive steps to prevent abusive behavior. This knowledge can also inform policy and practice, leading to the implementation of stronger protections for vulnerable individuals and increased accountability for abusive behavior.

Unlike many books on social care that focus on the values and behaviors that employees should follow, this book takes a different approach. It explores the values and traits that should be recognized and eliminated from the social care system, such as abuse and neglect. I recognize that this subject matter may be difficult, but it is essential reading for anyone working in or concerned about the welfare of vulnerable individuals in the social care system.

My goal with this book is to shine a light on the disturbing reality of abuse within the social care system and provide insights and recommendations for preventing and addressing abusive behavior. I emphasize the need for greater accountability and transparency within the system, as well as the importance of recognizing and addressing abusive behavior when it occurs.

I understand that this book may not be for everyone, and some readers may find it challenging or uncomfortable to read. However, I believe it is an important contribution to the discussion of abuse within the social care system. It provides a sobering reminder of the ongoing challenges facing the system and the need for continued efforts to protect the welfare of vulnerable individuals. I hope that readers will approach this book with an open mind and a willingness to confront the difficult subject matter it covers.

INTRODUCTION

Abuse is a significant problem in adult social care. It is estimated that around 1.5 million people in the UK use adult social care services, and a significant number of these individuals are vulnerable to abuse. According to a survey conducted by the Care Quality Commission (CQC) in 2019, 39% of care homes in England did not meet the required standards in relation to safety.

Abuse can take many forms, including physical, emotional, sexual, and financial abuse. It can occur in a variety of settings, including care homes, hospitals, and the individual's own home. The perpetrators of abuse can be family members, care workers, or other individuals with access to vulnerable adults.

There are several reasons why abuse is prevalent in adult social care. Firstly, many vulnerable adults are isolated and dependent on others for their care, which can make them more susceptible to abuse. Additionally, care workers may be poorly trained and underpaid, which can lead to high turnover rates and a lack of continuity of care. This can make it easier for perpetrators to abuse vulnerable adults without being detected.

Furthermore, there may be a culture of

indifference towards abuse in some care settings, where staff may turn a blind eye to abuse or fail to report it due to a fear of reprisals or a lack of support.

It is essential to raise awareness of the issue of abuse in adult social care and to provide adequate training and support for care workers to prevent and respond to abuse effectively. This includes providing training on safeguarding, promoting a culture of openness and accountability, and ensuring that care workers are adequately remunerated and valued for their work. By addressing the underlying factors that contribute to abuse in adult social care, we can help to ensure that vulnerable adults receive the care and support they need in a safe and compassionate environment.

There have been several high-profile instances of abuse in social care, both in the UK and globally, which have resulted in investigations and inquiries into the findings.

One notable example is the Winterbourne View Hospital scandal in 2011, in which an undercover investigation by the BBC's Panorama program exposed the abuse of vulnerable adults with learning disabilities and autism by staff at the hospital. The findings revealed a culture of abuse and neglect, including physical and psychological abuse, financial exploitation, and over-medication. The inquiry led to the closure of the hospital, criminal convictions for some staff members, and a government review of care for people with learning disabilities.

Another high-profile example is the Mid Staffordshire NHS Foundation Trust scandal in the UK, in which an independent inquiry revealed serious failings in care for patients, including neglect, inadequate care, and poor standards of hygiene. The findings of the inquiry revealed a culture of secrecy and defensiveness within the organization, and a lack of accountability for poor care. The inquiry led to major reforms in healthcare regulation and a renewed focus on patient safety and quality of care.

Globally, there have been instances of abuse in social care in other countries, such as the scandal at the nursing home in Quebec, Canada, where residents were found to have been neglected and mistreated by staff. The findings led to an inquiry and the introduction of new regulations and standards for care homes.

These high-profile instances of abuse in social care highlight the need for robust safeguarding measures and a culture of accountability and transparency in care settings. They also demonstrate the importance of rigorous regulation and inspection to ensure that care providers are delivering high-quality and compassionate care to vulnerable adults and children.

The unwillingness of people and organizations to

acknowledge, recognize, or address the abuse of adults in social care has been a major issue in many countries. There are several reasons why this is the case.

Firstly, many people believe that abuse in social care settings is rare or even non-existent, and that allegations of abuse are often exaggerated or false. This belief can make it difficult for individuals to recognize abuse when it occurs, and can lead to a culture of silence and denial around the issue.

Secondly, many people may be reluctant to report abuse because they fear retribution or retaliation from the abuser or the organization. This can be especially true for vulnerable adults who may be dependent on their abuser for care and support.

Thirdly, there may be systemic issues within social care organizations that make it difficult to identify and address abuse. This can include a lack of training or resources, a culture of secrecy or protectionism, and a failure to implement effective policies and procedures for reporting and investigating abuse.

There have been many high-profile instances of abuse in social care, which have highlighted the need for greater awareness, accountability, and action..

Subtle abuse refers to the kind of abuse that is

not easily detectable and often goes unnoticed. It is often more difficult to recognize than physical abuse, but can be just as damaging to the victim's mental and emotional wellbeing. Subtle abuse can take many forms, including emotional manipulation, psychological control, and financial exploitation.

One common example of subtle abuse is gaslighting, which involves manipulating someone into questioning their own perception of reality. This can involve denying or minimizing the abuse, making the victim feel as though they are crazy or overreacting. Another example of subtle abuse is isolation, where the abuser seeks to cut off the victim from their social support network, making it more difficult for them to seek help or escape the situation.

Subtle abuse can be particularly prevalent in social care settings, where the power dynamic between the caregiver and the client can create an environment that is ripe for abuse. Caregivers may use their position of authority to exert control over their clients, whether through emotional manipulation, financial exploitation, or other means.

One of the challenges with addressing subtle abuse is that it can be difficult to detect, particularly if the victim is not able to speak up or does not recognize the abuse themselves. It is important for caregivers and social care organizations to be vigilant and to create systems and processes that help to prevent and identify subtle abuse. This might include training programs for caregivers to recognize and prevent subtle abuse, as well as regular check-ins with clients to ensure their wellbeing and safety.

It is important for those working in social care to familiarize themselves with the techniques used by abusers, the unintentional abuser, and the psychology of abuse for several reasons.

Firstly, understanding the techniques used by abusers can help those working in social care to recognize the signs of abuse more easily. This can be particularly important in cases of subtle abuse, where the abuse may be difficult to detect. By being familiar with the various tactics that abusers may use, such as gaslighting, coercion, or isolation, social care workers can be better equipped to identify instances of abuse and take appropriate action to protect vulnerable adults.

Secondly, it is important for social care workers to be aware of unintentional abuse. Unintentional abuse can occur when a caregiver or social care worker unintentionally causes harm or distress to a vulnerable adult, often due to a lack of knowledge, skills, or resources. By understanding the potential causes of unintentional abuse, social care workers can take steps to prevent it from occurring, such as providing additional training or resources to staff.

Finally, understanding the psychology of abuse can help social care workers to provide more effective support and care to vulnerable adults. By understanding the dynamics of abuse, such as the power imbalance between the abuser and the victim, social care workers can provide more tailored and effective support to help victims of abuse to recover and heal.

In summary, familiarizing oneself with the techniques used by abusers, unintentional abuse, and the psychology of abuse can help those working in social care to identify instances of abuse more easily, prevent unintentional harm, and provide more effective support to vulnerable adults who have experienced abuse.

"Subtle Abuse in Adult Social Care," we will delve into various topics that pertain to abuse, in order to gain a deeper understanding of its intricate nature. Through the course of this book, we will provide an overview of the history of abuse and discuss the intention and psychology behind it, with a specific focus on how it is manifested in the context of adult social care. We will also examine notable scandals that have shaken the social care industry and explore the daunting challenges faced by whistleblowers who try to report abuse. To add depth to our discussion, we will provide firsthand accounts of individuals who have experienced and reported abuse in the context of adult social care.

Our goal is to raise awareness of the complex and often subtle nature of abuse in social care and provide guidance on how to identify and prevent it. By covering these topics, we hope to provide valuable insights and knowledge to individuals who work in or are affected by adult social care. Through this book, we aim to highlight the importance of creating safe and respectful environments for all individuals, particularly those who are most vulnerable.

HISTORY OF ABUSE

Throughout ancient history, vulnerable adults have been subject to abuse, neglect, and mistreatment. The poor, physically disabled, neurologically disabled, and those with psychiatric conditions have all been particularly vulnerable to mistreatment due to social stigmas and a lack of resources and support.

In ancient Greece, those with physical disabilities were often left to die on mountaintops or in other desolate areas. They were confined to institutions or left to fend for themselves on the streets. They were seen as a drain on resources and a burden to society. Some were even used as entertainment, forced to perform in public as a form of amusement.

In ancient Rome, people with physical disabilities were often viewed as objects of ridicule and were subjected to harsh treatment. Some were even used as gladiators, forced to fight to the death in front of crowds for the entertainment of others. Infanticide was also common, particularly for those with disabilities or born into poverty. In ancient Rome, slaves and the poor were subjected to abuse and mistreatment by those in power. Those with mental illness were often chained and confined to unsanitary living conditions.

The 1st century was a time of significant scientific and cultural change, but it was also a time of great difficulty for many disabled individuals. In general, people with disabilities in the 1st century were often marginalized, excluded from mainstream society, and subject to negative attitudes and beliefs. One factor that contributed to the poor treatment of disabled individuals in the 1st century was the lack of scientific understanding of disability. Many people believed that disabilities were caused by supernatural forces, such as curses or divine punishment, rather than by physical or environmental factors. This belief system often led to disabled individuals being ostracized or even persecuted, as they were viewed as being cursed or sinful.

In addition to these cultural and social factors, religious laws and traditions also played a significant role in worsening the plight of disabled individuals. For example, in Hebrew law, people with certain disabilities were considered unclean and were excluded from certain religious practices and rituals. This exclusion extended to people with physical disabilities, such as those with leprosy, as well as to those with mental health issues, such as those with epilepsy or schizophrenia.

The Roman Empire, which dominated much of the Mediterranean world in the 1st century, also had a complex relationship with disabled individuals.

While the empire did provide some forms of support and care for disabled individuals, such as medical treatment and financial assistance, disabled individuals were also subject to negative attitudes and beliefs. For example, in Roman law, children with disabilities could be abandoned or left to die if their parents deemed them to be unfit for survival.

Despite these challenges, disabled individuals in the 1st century also had access to systems of support and care, albeit limited by modern standards. For example, family members or other caregivers provided care and support, while religious institutions or charitable organizations sometimes provided assistance. However, the stigma and discrimination associated with disability often made it difficult for disabled individuals to access these support systems or to live fulfilling lives.

During the Middle Ages, individuals with disabilities were often viewed as being under the influence of demons and subjected to exorcisms or other cruel treatments. Those with mental illness were often accused of witchcraft and subjected to torture and execution. Throughout history, people with disabilities have been particularly vulnerable to accusations of witchcraft, often facing severe persecution and even death as a result. The accusations of witchcraft were often used as a means of scapegoating individuals who were seen as "other" or "different" and who could not defend themselves against these charges. In many cases, the accusations were based on superstition, fear, or prejudice, rather than any actual evidence of wrongdoing.

The plight of people with disabilities who were accused of witchcraft was particularly severe, as their disabilities often made them more vulnerable to the accusations and less able to defend themselves. In many cases, individuals with disabilities were accused of witchcraft because their disabilities were seen as evidence of a demonic possession or a curse. They were often subjected to brutal torture and interrogation in order to force them to confess to the accusations, even though they were often innocent.

The accusations of witchcraft also provided a benefit to their accusers, who could use the accusations as a means of gaining power or wealth. Accusers could benefit financially by seizing the property or assets of the accused, or by charging fees for their services as "witch-hunters." Additionally, the accusations of witchcraft often served to reinforce existing power structures, allowing the accusers to maintain their position of authority.

This can be compared to financial abuse, which is a form of exploitation that often targets vulnerable individuals such as people with disabilities or the elderly. Financial abuse involves using deceit or coercion to gain control over an individual's finances, often with the goal of enriching the abuser. Financial abusers may use tactics such as stealing money or assets, manipulating the individual into giving them access to their financial resources, or exploiting their trust or dependence. Like the accusations of witchcraft, financial abuse can have devastating consequences for the victim, who may be left without resources or means of support. Financial abuse can also reinforce existing power structures, allowing the abuser to maintain control over the victim and perpetuate their abuse.

In more recent history, the treatment of vulnerable adults has also been marked by abuse and mistreatment. In the 19th and early 20th centuries, those with mental illness were often confined to asylums and subjected to inhumane living conditions and treatments. Those with physical disabilities were often institutionalized and treated as objects of curiosity rather than human beings. The derogatory term of 'freak' was applied to people with deformities which was exacerbated by the invention of 'Freak shows.' These were a popular form of entertainment in the 19th and early 20th centuries featuring people with various physical and developmental disabilities, deformities, or medical conditions. These shows were exploitative and dehumanizing, with disabled individuals treated as objects of curiosity and spectacle rather than as fellow human beings. The experiences of disabled people who were displayed in freak shows were often traumatic and damaging to their physical and emotional well-being. One of the most significant challenges faced by people who were displayed in freak shows was the public scrutiny and ridicule they received. People with physical deformities or disabilities were often stared at and mocked by audiences who viewed them as freaks or monsters. This constant attention and humiliation could be incredibly damaging to an individual's self-esteem and mental health. Additionally, many people who were displayed in freak shows were forced to perform in ways that were physically demanding or painful. For example, some performers with physical disabilities were required to walk on their hands or contort their bodies in unnatural ways for the entertainment of audiences. Others were subjected to painful medical treatments or surgeries in order to make their deformities more pronounced. The conditions in which performers in freak shows were housed and cared for were poor as well. Many were kept in cramped quarters or makeshift tents and were not provided with adequate food, water, or medical care. They were also subject to exploitation by show managers and promoters, who often took a significant portion of their earnings and provided them with little or no financial support.

Finding documentation about the abuse of

disabled people from history can be challenging due to a number of factors. Disability has historically been stigmatized, and disabled people have been marginalized and excluded from society. This means that their experiences and perspectives have often been overlooked or actively suppressed in historical documentation.

One reason why it is difficult to find documentation about the abuse of disabled people from history is the lack of institutional accountability. In the past, institutions such as asylums and almshouses were largely self-regulating, and there was little oversight or accountability for the treatment of disabled people within them. This made it easy for abuse to occur and go unreported or undocumented.

Another reason why it is difficult to find documentation about the abuse of disabled people from history is the selective nature of historical documentation. Historians and archivists have often focused on the perspectives of dominant groups in society, such as white men, and have overlooked the experiences of marginalized groups, including disabled people.

In addition, the documentation of abuse from history is often hidden or obscured by other historical events or narratives. For example, the history of colonialism, slavery, and genocide has often been presented as a heroic narrative of exploration, civilization, and progress, rather than as a history of exploitation, violence, and oppression.

In contrast to the difficulties of finding documentation of abuse from history, the current media-filled world provides a platform for people to speak out about abuse and to hold perpetrators accountable. Social media, in particular, has given a voice to marginalized groups and has helped to expose instances of abuse and neglect.

The #MeToo movement, for example, has brought attention to the prevalence of sexual harassment and assault, and has led to increased awareness and action to address these issues. Similarly, the disability rights movement has been instrumental in bringing attention to the abuse and neglect of disabled people, and in advocating for greater legal protections and social support.

The case of Winterbourne, a residential care home where residents with learning disabilities were subject to physical and emotional abuse, highlights the hidden conditions that many people with disabilities have coped with throughout human history.
The abuse at Winterbourne, which came to light in 2011, involved staff members physically assaulting residents, forcing them to take cold showers, and taunting them with insults and threats. The abuse was carried out in secret, away

from the view of family members and other outside observers.

This case is just one example of the many instances of abuse and neglect that have occurred throughout human history, often in secret and out of the public eye. In many cases, people with disabilities have been institutionalized or otherwise isolated from society, making it easy for abuse to occur without detection or intervention.

The history of institutionalization and segregation of people with disabilities dates back centuries, and was often driven by a desire to isolate and control individuals who were seen as a burden or a threat to society. As a result, people with disabilities were often hidden away in institutions such as asylums or almshouses, where they were subject to neglect, abuse, and exploitation.

The case of Winterbourne highlights the ongoing challenges faced by people with disabilities in accessing safe and supportive care and support. It also underscores the importance of shining a light on the hidden conditions that people with disabilities have faced throughout history.

While the exposure of abuse and neglect is an important step towards ensuring the safety and well-being of people with disabilities, it is also important to address the root causes of these issues. This includes challenging the stigma and discrimination faced by people with disabilities, promoting greater social inclusion and participation, and providing accessible and appropriate care and support.

Finding documentation about the abuse of disabled people from history can be difficult due to a range of social, institutional, and historical factors. However, the current media-filled world provides new opportunities for people to speak out about abuse and to hold perpetrators accountable. It is essential that we continue to shine a light on the experiences of marginalized groups and work towards a more just and equitable society.

THE FIRST CAMPAIGNERS
FOR HUMAN RIGHTS

*The Society for the Reformation of Manners and Sir
Matthew Hale*

Witch hunting, from today's perspective, would be considered a form of human rights abuse. This is because witch hunts involve the persecution and punishment of individuals based on unfounded and often superstitious beliefs and accusations. These accusations were often made without evidence or due process, and the accused were frequently subjected to torture, imprisonment, and even execution.

Witch hunts also often targeted marginalized and vulnerable groups, such as women, the elderly, and those with disabilities or mental health issues. These individuals were particularly vulnerable to accusations of witchcraft and were more likely to be subjected to the most severe forms of punishment.

There were often financial incentives for accusing someone of being a witch. These incentives varied depending on the specific context and location, but they typically involved some form of payment or reward for reporting a suspected witch to the authorities.

In some cases, the reward for accusing someone of witchcraft came in the form of a monetary payment or a share of the accused person's property. For example, in England, a law was passed in 1563 that allowed anyone who convicted a witch to claim one-third of the accused person's property. This law created a financial incentive for people to make false accusations of witchcraft, as it allowed them to profit from the conviction and punishment of the accused. Furthermore, witch hunts were often carried out by those in positions of power, such as religious leaders or government officials, who used their authority to perpetrate acts of violence and oppression against those they perceived as threats. This abuse of power further compounded the injustices and harms inflicted upon the accused.

The Society for the Reformation of Manners and Sir Matthew Hale were two prominent forces in the campaign to end the practice of witch-hunting in England. Their work helped to raise awareness of the injustice of witch hunts and played a key role in convincing Parliament to pass the Witchcraft Act of 1735, which put an end to the practice of witch-hunting in England.

The Society for the Reformation of Manners was a group of English intellectuals, including theologians, philosophers and members of the Royal Society, such as John Locke who were concerned about the growing influence of immorality and vice in English society. The group believed that moral decline was a major cause of social problems and that a more virtuous and godly society was needed to address these issues. As part of their efforts to promote moral reform, the Society focused on a range of issues, including public drunkenness, prostitution, gambling, and swearing. They also campaigned against the practice of witch-hunting, which they saw as a particularly egregious example of the dangers of superstition and fanaticism.

Sir Matthew Hale was a prominent English judge and legal scholar who played a key role in the campaign to end witch-hunting. He was skeptical of the claims made by witch-hunters and argued that the evidence used to convict accused witches was often unreliable and that the punishments meted out to them were cruel and disproportionate. In his writings and advocacy, Hale helped to raise awareness of the injustice of witch hunts and played a pivotal role in convincing Parliament to pass the Witchcraft Act of 1735. Together, the Society for the Reformation of Manners and Sir Matthew Hale helped to shift public attitudes towards witchcraft and played a key role in the eventual passage of the Witchcraft Act of 1735. This law repealed the Witchcraft Act of 1542 and made it a crime to claim that any person had magical powers or was guilty of practicing witchcraft. The law helped to put an end to the practice of witch-hunting in England and marked a significant turning point in attitudes towards witchcraft.

The influence of the Society for the Reformation of Manners and Sir Matthew Hale in the campaign against witch-hunting was driven by their shared commitment to justice, fairness, and evidence-based reasoning. They saw the witch-hunts as a form of injustice that violated the basic rights and dignity of accused witches, and they worked tirelessly to promote a more rational and fair approach to the investigation of witchcraft accusations. Today, their legacy lives on as a reminder of the importance of justice, morality, and social activism in promoting human rights and social progress. Their work helped to put an end to the practice of witch-hunting in England, and their advocacy continues to inspire those who seek to promote justice and human dignity in the modern world.

Reasons for outlawing abuse.

Enlightenment ideas: During the Enlightenment, there was a growing emphasis on reason, science, and rationality. Many Enlightenment thinkers rejected superstition and believed that people should be judged based on evidence and reason, rather than superstition and hearsay. This led to a questioning of the witch-hunting beliefs and practices.

The rise of the scientific method: The scientific method, which emphasizes experimentation, observation, and evidence-based reasoning, also helped to discredit many of the claims of witch-hunters. As people became more educated and more skilled at using scientific methods, they were better able to debunk the myths and superstitions surrounding witchcraft.

Changes in legal systems: As countries became more organized and centralized, legal systems began to develop that were less reliant on local or religious authorities. This helped to curb the power of witch-hunters and make it more difficult for them to prosecute individuals without due process.

Increasing skepticism: As the practice of witch-hunting became more widespread, people became increasingly skeptical of its validity. They began to question the evidence used to convict accused witches and to challenge the motives of the witch-hunters themselves.

The values designed to protect vulnerable people were based on strengthening objectivity. Objective and scientific values have played a crucial role in protecting disabled people from societal prejudice and persecution by promoting evidence-based practices, objectivity, and equality. Scientific values have promoted evidence-based practices in healthcare, research, and other fields, which has led to the development of effective treatments and interventions that improve the lives of people with disabilities. This has helped reduce stigma and discrimination against disabled people by increasing understanding and acceptance of their needs and experiences.

Objectivity is a fundamental principle of scientific inquiry, which has helped to challenge harmful stereotypes and biases about disabilities. By promoting a rigorous examination of evidence, scientific values can provide a more accurate and nuanced understanding of the experiences and needs of disabled people, which can help to reduce negative attitudes and assumptions. Objective and scientific values have also promoted equality by prioritizing equal access to education, employment, and other opportunities for people with disabilities. By relying on empirical data and rigorous testing, objective and scientific values can help identify and address barriers to access and provide evidence-based solutions to promote inclusion and equality. Moreover, objective and scientific values have played a critical role in promoting ethical behavior and responsible decision-making. By prioritizing ethical principles such as informed consent, confidentiality, and the protection of vulnerable populations, objective and scientific values can help ensure that disabled people are treated with the respect and dignity they deserve.

THE FIRST CARE INSTITUTIONS

Almshouses

However, the first formal institutions specifically designed for the care of people with disabilities were established in Europe during the Middle Ages. These institutions, known as almshouses or hospitals, were typically run by religious orders and provided basic care and shelter to disabled individuals, as well as to the poor and elderly.

The concept of almshouses can be traced back to the early Christian church, which established monastic communities to provide care and support for the sick and needy. These communities were self-sufficient, and relied on donations from wealthy patrons to fund their operations. Over time, these monastic communities evolved into the first almshouses, which were established throughout Europe in the 12th and 13th centuries.

Almshouses were typically run by religious orders, such as monks or nuns, and provided a range of services to their residents. These services included shelter, food, medical care, and education. Many almshouses also had strict rules and regulations governing behavior and daily routines, and residents were often required to attend church services and other religious ceremonies.

In many cases, almshouses were the only option available to people with disabilities who had been abandoned by their families or were unable to care for themselves. In many cases, almshouses were overcrowded and understaffed, with residents living in squalid conditions and receiving little or no medical care or rehabilitation services. The lack of resources and training often led to staff members mistreating and neglecting residents. There were numerous reports of physical and emotional abuse, including beatings, restraints, and verbal abuse.

One of the most troubling aspects of life in almshouses was the social isolation that residents experienced. Residents were often separated from their families and friends, and had little contact with the outside world. This isolation could exacerbate existing mental health conditions and contribute to the development of new ones. Residents with physical and mental disabilities were particularly vulnerable to neglect and abuse. Many almshouses were not equipped to provide specialized care for individuals with disabilities, and staff members often lacked the training and resources necessary to care for these residents. As a result, many residents with disabilities were subjected to harsh living conditions and mistreatment.

The abuses that occurred in almshouses were not unique to any particular time or place. Throughout history, almshouses have been associated with neglect and abuse, and the experiences of residents in these institutions have been a source of shame and controversy.

Despite these challenges, almshouses played an important role in the development of care institutions for people with disabilities. They provided a basic model for the provision of shelter and support to vulnerable populations, and many of the principles that were established in almshouses - such as the importance of community and social support - continue to inform the care of individuals with disabilities today.

Asylums

The purpose of an asylum is to provide a safe and controlled environment for individuals who are unable to care for themselves due to mental illness, physical disabilities, or other conditions that leave them vulnerable. These institutions are intended to provide basic care and support to vulnerable populations, with a focus on developing specialized care and treatment for patients. However, the word "asylum" has become stigmatized over time, with negative connotations associated with institutionalization, social isolation, and the mistreatment of patients. This stigma has arisen due to the history of abuse and neglect that occurred in some asylums, as well as a broader cultural association between mental illness and stigma.

Asylums were first introduced in Europe in the 18th century as a way to care for the vulnerable populations who were unable to care for themselves, including individuals with mental illness, physical disabilities, and other conditions that left them unable to live independently.

The first asylums were established in Europe in the 18th century, with the earliest institutions often run by religious orders or other charitable organizations. These institutions were intended to provide basic care and support to individuals with mental illness or other disabilities, but they were often overcrowded and understaffed, and residents were subject to neglect and abuse.

In the United States, the first public mental hospital was established in 1773 in Williamsburg, Virginia, which was intended to provide care and treatment for individuals with mental illness. However, like in Europe, conditions in early asylums were often harsh, and residents lived in squalid conditions with little access to medical care or rehabilitation services.

Asylums played an important role in the development of care for individuals with mental illness and other disabilities. They provided a controlled environment for those deemed a danger to themselves or others, and many institutions focused on developing specialized care and treatment for patients. However, the history of asylums is also marked by controversy and criticism. Many institutions were overcrowded and understaffed, with residents subjected to neglect, abuse, and social isolation. The overuse of institutionalization in the 20th century led to a movement towards community-based care and deinstitutionalization, with the belief that individuals with mental illness were better served by living in the community with access to appropriate medical and social support

The late 19th century saw significant advances in the understanding and treatment of neurological disabilities, including conditions such as epilepsy, cerebral palsy, and traumatic brain injury. These advances were driven by developments in medical science, as well as a growing recognition of the importance of specialized care and support for individuals with neurological disabilities. One of the key developments during this period was the introduction of anti-epileptic drugs, which were first developed in the 1860s. These medications, including phenobarbital and bromides, were effective in reducing the frequency and severity of seizures in individuals with epilepsy. This allowed many patients to live more independent lives and to participate more fully in their communities.

Another important development was the use of physical therapy and rehabilitation to improve the function and mobility of individuals with neurological disabilities. This approach involved a combination of exercise, massage, and other techniques designed to improve muscle strength and flexibility, as well as improve the functioning of the nervous system. In addition, the late 19th century saw the development of specialized institutions for individuals with neurological disabilities, including hospitals, schools, and residential facilities. These institutions provided specialized care and support for individuals with conditions such as cerebral palsy and traumatic brain injury, and often incorporated physical therapy and other forms of rehabilitation into their treatment programs. Despite these advances, many individuals with neurological disabilities continued to face significant challenges in accessing appropriate care and support. Stigma and discrimination were still common, and many individuals were denied the opportunity to live full and independent lives. However, the developments of the late 19th century laid the groundwork for further advances in the understanding and treatment of neurological disabilities in the 20th century, and provided hope for individuals and families affected by these conditions.

The transition from asylums to hospitals for

people with physical and learning disabilities began in the mid-20th century, as part of a broader movement towards deinstitutionalization and community-based care.

Prior to this transition, individuals with physical and learning disabilities were often housed in large institutions known as asylums or almshouses. These institutions were often overcrowded and understaffed, and residents were subject to neglect and abuse.

In the mid-20th century, a number of factors led to a movement towards community-based care and support for individuals with physical and learning disabilities. These factors included advances in medical and social support, as well as concerns about the overuse of institutionalization and the poor quality of care in asylums. As a result, many institutions began to shift towards a hospital-based model of care. Hospitals were seen as a way to provide more specialized and targeted care for individuals with physical and learning disabilities, while also allowing for greater opportunities for community integration and participation. The transition from asylums to hospitals was not without its challenges. Many hospitals were initially designed to provide acute care and treatment, rather than long-term care and support. As a result, patients often faced shorter hospital stays and more frequent transitions between hospitals and community-based settings. In addition, the transition from asylums to hospitals was often accompanied by a lack of funding and resources for community-based care and support. Many individuals with physical and learning disabilities faced significant barriers in accessing the services and support they needed to live full and independent lives.

SUPPORT TO LIVE IN
THE COMMUNITY

The UK's transition from institutionalized care to supported living in the community has been a gradual process that began in the mid-20th century and continues to this day. The transition has been driven by a number of factors, including advances in medical and social support, concerns about the overuse of institutionalization, and a growing recognition of the importance of individualized and community-based care.

The movement towards community-based care began in the 1950s and 1960s, when a number of institutions were closed or downsized in response to concerns about the quality of care and the rights of individuals with disabilities. This led to the development of a range of community-based services and supports, including group homes, day programs, and other forms of supported living.

In the 1980s and 1990s, the UK government began to focus more explicitly on promoting community-based care and support for individuals with disabilities. This included the introduction of legislation such as the Community Care Act 1990, which emphasized the importance of individualized care and support in the community.

Today, the focus is on providing a range of community-based services and supports that allow individuals with disabilities to live full and independent lives. This includes the provision of housing, employment support, social and recreational activities, and other forms of support tailored to the individual needs and circumstances of each person.

The transition from institutionalized care to supported living in the community has been accompanied by a number of challenges, including the need for increased funding and resources for community-based services, as well as the need for more widespread education and awareness about the benefits of community-based care. Despite these challenges, the movement towards community-based care and support has led to significant improvements in the quality of life for individuals with disabilities in the UK. By focusing on individualized and community-based care, the UK has been able to provide more targeted and effective services and supports, while also promoting greater social inclusion and participation for individuals with disabilities.

The change from hospital institutionalized care to community-based support was gradually introduced due to a number of reasons. These include:

Human Rights: One of the main reasons for the change was the recognition of the rights of people with disabilities to live independently in their communities. Institutionalized care was seen as a violation of these rights, as it often involved isolation, segregation, and a lack of autonomy and choice.

Quality of Life: Community-based care was seen as offering a better quality of life for people with disabilities. In a community setting, people with disabilities can be involved in daily activities, have access to social and recreational activities, and maintain relationships with family and friends. This helps to promote their mental and emotional well-being.

Cost-Effectiveness: Community-based care is generally less expensive than institutionalized care. This is because community-based care requires less staff, infrastructure, and resources. Community-based care also helps to reduce hospitalizations and emergency room visits, which can be costly for both individuals and the healthcare system.

Advances in Medical and Social Support: Advances in medical and social support have made it possible for people with disabilities to live independently in the community. Assistive technology, adaptive housing, and community-based services and supports have made it possible for people with disabilities to manage their own lives and participate in their communities.

Deinstitutionalization: The movement towards deinstitutionalization was a major driving force behind the change from hospital institutionalized care to community-based support. This movement was based on the belief that people with disabilities should be integrated into their communities and have access to the same rights and opportunities as everyone else.

In conclusion, the change from hospital institutionalized care to community-based support was driven by a number of factors, including the recognition of human rights, the desire for a better quality of life, cost-effectiveness, advances in medical and social support, and the movement towards deinstitutionalization. These factors have led to significant improvements in the lives of people with disabilities, and have helped to promote greater social inclusion and participation.

THE DANGER STILL EXISTS

The inevitability of abuse in today's care services is a sad reality, and it often stays hidden from scrutiny due to a number of complex factors. While the majority of care providers are dedicated to providing high-quality care to those in need, the reality is that instances of abuse do occur, and they can have devastating consequences for those affected.

One of the main reasons why abuse can occur in care services is the lack of oversight and regulation. Many care providers operate with minimal supervision, and there is often little accountability for those who engage in abusive behavior. This can create an environment in which abuse can occur without detection or intervention. Another factor contributing to the inevitability of abuse is the power dynamic that exists between care providers and those in their care. Care providers often have significant power and control over the lives of their clients, which can make it difficult for clients to report abuse or seek help. This can be especially true for those with disabilities or mental health issues, who may be particularly vulnerable to abuse. In addition, the complexity of care services can make it difficult for abuse to be detected. Many care services are provided in private homes, which can make it difficult for outside observers to monitor care providers and ensure that abuse is not taking place. Similarly, the variety of services provided by care providers can make it challenging for regulators to maintain effective oversight. Despite these challenges, there are steps that can be taken to address the inevitability of abuse in care services. These include strengthening regulation and oversight, improving the training and support provided to care providers, and empowering clients and their families to report abuse and seek help. It is also important to recognize that abuse can have profound effects on those who experience it, and that it is essential to provide support and resources to those affected. This includes counseling and therapy, as well as legal and advocacy services. Ultimately, addressing the inevitability of abuse in care services requires a multifaceted approach that involves all stakeholders, including care providers, regulators, clients, and their families. By working together to address this critical issue, we can help to ensure that those in need receive the high-quality care and support they deserve, and that instances of abuse are detected and addressed as quickly as possible.

WINTERBOURNE VIEW

Winterbourne is a name that will forever be associated with one of the most shocking cases of abuse and neglect of vulnerable adults in modern history. The events at Winterbourne, a residential care home in South Gloucestershire, UK, exposed the horrors that can occur when those entrusted with the care of vulnerable adults betray that trust and inflict unimaginable harm.

The story of Winterbourne began to emerge in 2011, when an undercover reporter for the BBC's Panorama program began investigating reports of abuse at the care home. What he found was beyond disturbing: staff members physically and emotionally abusing residents, subjecting them to beatings, forced cold showers, and verbal taunts and insults. The abuse was captured on video, and the footage was aired on national television, sparking public outrage and calls for action. The abuse had been carried out in secret, away from the view of family members and outside authorities. The residents, who were largely nonverbal and had limited communication skills, were unable to report the abuse themselves. The story of Winterbourne is a tragic reminder of the vulnerability of people with learning disabilities, and of the importance of holding care providers accountable for the safety and well-being of their clients. It sparked a national conversation about the need for greater protection and oversight, and led to reforms aimed at ensuring that people with learning disabilities are treated with dignity, respect, and compassion. The aftermath of the Winterbourne scandal was far-reaching. The owners of the care home were prosecuted and sentenced to lengthy prison terms, and the Care Quality Commission (CQC), the UK's regulatory body for health and social care, faced criticism for failing to detect the abuse sooner. The incident led to a public inquiry and a review of the regulatory framework for residential care homes. The story of Winterbourne is a stark reminder that abuse and neglect of vulnerable adults can occur in any care setting, and that it is essential to remain vigilant and hold care providers accountable for their actions. It is also a testament to the power of the media in exposing abuses and catalyzing change, and to the courage of whistleblowers who speak out against wrongdoing. The legacy of Winterbourne will continue to shape the landscape of care for vulnerable adults for years to come. The abuse that took place at Winterbourne care home, which was exposed by an undercover reporter for the BBC's Panorama program, was truly shocking and disturbing. The footage captured by the reporter revealed a litany of abuses and neglect inflicted on the vulnerable residents of the care home. The staff members at

Winterbourne were seen physically and emotionally abusing the residents, subjecting them to beatings, forced cold showers, and verbal taunts and insults. Some of the most egregious abuses included:

- Residents being hit with shoes, chairs, and other objects.
- Residents were pinned to the ground and restrained in a way that restricted their breathing.
- Residents being dragged, pushed, and kicked.
- Residents being threatened with violence and taunted with cruel and offensive language.
- Residents being force-fed medication and physically restrained during medical procedures.
- Residents are left to sit in soiled clothing and bedding for extended periods of time.
- Residents being denied food and water as a form of punishment.

These abuses were carried out over a period of several months, with little or no oversight or intervention from outside authorities. The residents were largely nonverbal and had limited communication skills, which made it difficult for them to report the abuse themselves. Family members of the residents were largely unaware of the abuse, as the staff at Winterbourne had gone to great lengths to conceal their actions.

The abuse that took place at Winterbourne was not only physically and emotionally damaging to the residents, but also a violation of their human rights and dignity. The incident sparked a national conversation about the need for greater protection and oversight for vulnerable adults in residential care homes, and led to a public inquiry and a review of the regulatory framework for care homes.

The legacy of Winterbourne serves as a reminder that abuse and neglect of vulnerable adults can occur in any care setting, and that it is essential to remain vigilant and hold care providers accountable for their actions. It also highlights the importance of whistleblowers who are brave enough to speak out against wrongdoing and the power of the media in exposing abuses and catalyzing change.

Whistleblowers play a critical role in exposing abuses and wrongdoings, particularly in the care industry where vulnerable individuals may not be able to speak out for themselves. In the case of the Winterbourne scandal, the whistleblower who came forward faced a number of challenges and difficulties in reporting the abuse and bringing it to light. The whistleblower, Terry Bryan, was a former senior nurse at Winterbourne care home who had become increasingly alarmed by the abuse he was witnessing. He tried to raise his concerns with the management of the care home and with the relevant authorities, but his complaints were ignored or dismissed. Bryan eventually contacted the Care Quality Commission (CQC), the UK's regulatory body for health and social care, and provided them with evidence of the abuse that was taking place at Winterbourne. However, the CQC failed to take any meaningful action, and the abuse continued unchecked for months.

It wasn't until an undercover reporter for the BBC's Panorama program infiltrated Winterbourne and captured footage of the abuse that the scandal finally came to light. Even then, the whistleblower faced backlash from the management of the care home, who accused him of breaching confidentiality and threatened legal action against him. The whistleblower in the Winterbourne scandal, Terry Bryan, must have felt a range of emotions during the course of his involvement in the case. As a former senior nurse at the care home, Bryan was deeply troubled by the abuse and neglect he witnessed and felt a sense of responsibility to do something about it. However, Bryan's attempts to raise his concerns with the management of the care home and with the relevant authorities were met with resistance and indifference. He must have felt frustrated and helpless at being unable to effect change or get anyone to take his concerns seriously.

Bryan's decision to contact the Care Quality Commission (CQC) and provide them with evidence of the abuse was likely a difficult one. He may have felt apprehensive about the potential consequences of speaking out, such as retaliation from the care home management or legal action against him. Despite these concerns, however, Bryan's commitment to exposing the abuse and protecting the vulnerable residents at Winterbourne drove him to take action. His decision to blow the whistle on the abuse was a brave and selfless one, and likely reflected a deep sense of moral conviction. Throughout the investigation and aftermath of the scandal, Bryan may have felt a range of emotions, including relief that the abuse had been exposed, frustration at the slow pace of progress in holding those responsible accountable, and a sense of satisfaction in knowing that his efforts had contributed to change and reform in the care industry.

The difficulties faced by whistleblowers like Terry Bryan highlight the challenges of speaking out against abuses and wrongdoings, particularly in cases where those in power may be resistant to change or accountability. Whistleblowers may face intimidation, retaliation, or even legal action, which can make it difficult for them to come forward and report abuses. However, the courage and determination of whistleblowers like Bryan can also serve as a powerful force for change. Their willingness to speak out and expose abuses can help to bring about accountability and reform, and ensure that vulnerable individuals are protected and cared for with dignity and respect. It is important that whistleblowers are supported and protected in their efforts to bring about change, and that their contributions are acknowledged and valued.

The staff and management of Winterbourne care home were held accountable for the abuses and neglect of the vulnerable residents in their care. Following the exposure of the abuse, the staff members involved were suspended and eventually dismissed from their positions. The management team, which included the owners of Winterbourne, faced criminal charges and were sentenced to prison terms ranging from two to three years for ill-treatment and wilful neglect of the residents under their care. In addition to the criminal charges, the staff and management of Winterbourne also faced civil lawsuits from the victims of the abuse and their families. The care home owners were ordered to pay significant compensation to the victims, as well as legal fees and other costs. The scandal resulted in a public inquiry and a review of the regulatory framework for residential care homes. The Care Quality Commission (CQC), the UK's regulatory body for health and social care, faced criticism for failing to detect the abuse sooner and underwent significant reforms in response to the scandal.

It is not clear why the abuse at Winterbourne went unnoticed for so long, but it is likely that a combination of factors contributed to this. These could include a lack of oversight and monitoring of the care home, a failure of regulatory bodies to detect the abuse, and a lack of whistleblower protections for those who might have been aware of the abuse but felt unable to come forward. The length of time that the abuse went on underscores the importance of robust safeguarding and monitoring procedures in care homes, as well as the need for mechanisms to detect and respond to incidents of abuse quickly and effectively. It also highlights the vital role that whistleblowers can play in exposing abuses and ensuring that vulnerable individuals are protected and cared for with dignity and respect.

While it is difficult to say how widespread this problem is, there are concerns that similar incidents of abuse and neglect may be occurring in other care homes, both in the UK and around the world. There are several reasons why this might be the case.

For one, care homes are often understaffed and under-resourced, which can lead to staff members feeling overwhelmed and unable to provide the level of care and attention that residents require. Additionally, the residents of care homes are often among the most vulnerable members of society, with limited communication skills and a reduced ability to report incidents of abuse or neglect.

Furthermore, there is a history of institutional abuse and neglect of people with disabilities and mental health issues, which suggests that such abuses may be deeply ingrained in some care systems. This can create a culture of silence and complicity, where staff members feel unable or unwilling to speak out against abuses they may witness.

The likelihood of abuse and neglect occurring in care homes underscores the need for greater oversight and regulation of these facilities, as well as the need for robust safeguarding and monitoring procedures. This includes ensuring that care home staff are appropriately trained and supported, and that whistleblowers are protected and encouraged to come forward with concerns.

Ultimately, preventing abuse and neglect in care homes requires a collective effort, involving care providers, regulatory bodies, policymakers, and society as a whole. It is important to remain vigilant and take action to address incidents of abuse or neglect when they are discovered, in order to ensure that vulnerable individuals receive the care and protection they deserve.

The aftermath of the Winterbourne scandal serves as a stark reminder of the importance of holding care providers accountable for the safety and well-being of their clients. The case highlights the vulnerability of people with learning disabilities and the importance of ensuring that they are treated with dignity, respect, and compassion. It also led to reforms aimed at improving oversight and regulation of residential care homes and ensuring that incidents of abuse and neglect are identified and addressed quickly and effectively.

WHALTON HALL

Whorlton Hall was a care home for adults with learning disabilities in County Durham, UK, which became embroiled in a scandal in 2019 after undercover footage revealed widespread abuse and mistreatment of residents by staff members.

The footage, captured by the BBC's Panorama program, showed staff members at Whorlton Hall assaulting, restraining, and verbally abusing residents, many of whom had limited communication skills and were unable to report the abuse themselves. The footage also showed staff members using derogatory and abusive language, referring to residents as "stupid" and "brain dead."

The abuse at Whorlton Hall care home, as captured by the BBC's Panorama program, involved a range of physical and verbal abuses towards vulnerable residents with learning disabilities. Some of the forms of abuse recorded at Whorlton Hall include:

Physical abuse: The footage showed staff members hitting, pushing, and slapping residents, as well as restraining them with excessive force. Punching and slapping: Staff members were recorded punching and slapping residents, often for no apparent reason.

1. Kicking and tripping: In some instances, staff members were recorded kicking or tripping residents, causing them to fall or lose their balance.

2. Restraint: Staff members at Whorlton Hall frequently restrained residents using excessive force, sometimes resulting in serious injuries. The footage showed residents being pinned to the ground or restrained with handcuffs, belts, or other restraints.

3. Rough handling: Staff members were also recorded roughly handling residents, such as pulling them by their arms or dragging them along the floor.

The physical abuse at Whorlton Hall was particularly disturbing given the vulnerability of the residents, many of whom had limited communication skills and were unable to report the abuse themselves. The abuses were a clear violation of the residents' human rights and dignity, and highlighted the importance of safeguarding and monitoring procedures in care homes.

Verbal abuse: Staff members were recorded using derogatory and abusive language towards residents, including using terms like "stupid," "idiot," and "brain dead." The verbal abuse captured on the undercover footage from Whorlton Hall care home was deeply distressing and highlighted the disrespect and lack of compassion shown towards vulnerable residents with learning disabilities. The footage showed staff members using derogatory and abusive language towards residents, often using terms like "stupid," "idiot," and "brain dead." Some of the specific instances of verbal abuse recorded at Whorlton Hall include:

1. **Mocking and taunting:** Staff members were recorded mocking and taunting residents, often in a cruel and degrading manner. For example, staff members were heard imitating the sounds made by residents or mocking their physical movements.

2. **Name-calling:** Staff members were also recorded calling residents derogatory names, using terms like "moron," "retard," and "dumbo."

3. **Threats:** In some instances, staff members were recorded threatening residents, using their power and authority to intimidate and control them. For example, staff members threatened to withhold food or water from residents or to use physical force against them.

The verbal abuse at Whorlton Hall was particularly concerning given the vulnerability of the residents and their limited ability to communicate or defend themselves. The use of derogatory and abusive language not only undermined the dignity and self-worth of the residents but also created a culture of disrespect and neglect within the care home.

The footage of the verbal abuse at Whorlton Hall was a stark reminder of the importance of treating vulnerable adults with respect, compassion, and dignity. It highlighted the need for better training and support for care home staff, as well as the importance of robust monitoring and oversight to ensure that abuses are identified and addressed quickly and effectively. The scandal also led to calls for greater accountability and regulation within the care home industry, to ensure that the needs and rights of vulnerable residents are prioritized and protected.

Emotional abuse: Residents were subjected to emotional abuse, such as being taunted or mocked by staff members, or being left alone and isolated for long periods of time.The emotional abuse captured on the undercover footage from Whorlton Hall care home was particularly concerning, as it involved a range of harmful behaviors that had a serious impact on the well-being and mental health of vulnerable residents with learning disabilities. The footage showed staff members subjecting residents to emotional abuse, such as taunting or mocking them, or leaving them alone and isolated for long periods of time. Some of the specific instances of emotional abuse recorded at Whorlton Hall include:

1. **Taunting and mocking:** Staff members were recorded taunting and mocking residents, often in a cruel and degrading manner. This included making fun of their physical appearance, imitating their speech or movements, or making derogatory comments about their behavior.

2. **Isolation:** Residents were also left alone and isolated for long periods of time, with little or no social interaction or stimulation. This led to feelings of loneliness, boredom, and despair, which in turn had a negative impact on their mental health and well-being.

3. **Neglect:** In some instances, emotional abuse also involved neglect, where staff members failed to provide the necessary care and support to residents. This included failing to help residents with basic tasks like bathing, dressing, or using the toilet, or ignoring their requests for assistance.

The emotional abuse at Whorlton Hall was particularly concerning given the vulnerability of the residents and their limited ability to communicate or defend themselves. The abuse had a serious impact on their mental health and well-being, and created an environment of fear and despair within the care home.

The footage of the emotional abuse at Whorlton Hall was a reminder of the importance of providing compassionate and respectful care to vulnerable adults with learning disabilities. It highlighted the need for better training and support for care home staff, as well as the importance of robust monitoring and oversight to ensure that abuses are identified and addressed quickly and effectively. The scandal also led to calls for greater accountability and regulation within the care home industry, to ensure that the needs and rights of vulnerable residents are prioritized and protected.

Neglect: The footage also showed instances of neglect, where staff members failed to provide adequate care and support to residents, such as failing to help them bathe or use the toilet. The neglect captured on the undercover footage from Whorlton Hall care home was particularly concerning, as it involved a range of harmful behaviors that had a serious impact on the health and well-being of vulnerable residents with learning disabilities. The footage showed staff members neglecting residents, such as failing to provide the necessary care and support to help them bathe, dress or use the toilet. Some of the specific instances of neglect recorded at Whorlton Hall include:

1. **Poor hygiene:** Staff members were recorded failing to help residents with basic hygiene needs, such as bathing, brushing their teeth or combing their hair. This led to a build-up of dirt, grime and unpleasant odors, which in turn had a negative impact on the mental health and self-esteem of residents.

2. **Inadequate nutrition:** Residents were also neglected in terms of their nutritional needs, with staff members failing to provide them with adequate food or drink. Some residents were observed eating food that was out of date or stale, while others were left without food or water for extended periods of time.

3. **Lack of medical attention:** In some instances, neglect also involved failing to provide residents with the necessary medical attention or treatment. This included failing to administer medication as prescribed, or failing to seek medical help when residents were clearly in

distress or experiencing pain.

The neglect at Whorlton Hall was particularly concerning given the vulnerability of the residents and their dependence on staff members for their basic needs. The neglect had a serious impact on the health and well-being of residents, and created an environment of neglect and indifference within the care home.

The footage of the neglect at Whorlton Hall was a reminder of the importance of providing adequate care and support to vulnerable adults with learning disabilities. It highlighted the need for better training and support for care home staff, as well as the importance of robust monitoring and oversight to ensure that abuses are identified and addressed quickly and effectively. The scandal also led to calls for greater accountability and regulation within the care home industry, to ensure that the needs and rights of vulnerable residents are prioritized and protected.

Financial abuse: There were also reports of financial abuse, where staff members stole money or possessions from residents. The financial abuse captured on the undercover footage from Whorlton Hall care home was particularly concerning, as it involved staff members exploiting vulnerable residents with learning disabilities for their own personal gain. The footage showed staff members stealing money or possessions from residents, which is a form of financial abuse. Some of the specific instances of financial abuse recorded at Whorlton Hall include:

1. **Stealing money:** Staff members were recorded stealing money from residents' wallets or purses, or taking cash that was meant for specific purposes like buying snacks or going on outings.

2. **Misusing bank cards:** In some instances, staff members were recorded misusing residents' bank cards, either by using them to withdraw money or by making unauthorized purchases.

3. **Stealing possessions:** Staff members were also recorded stealing possessions from residents, such as mobile phones, tablets or other personal items.

The financial abuse at Whorlton Hall was particularly concerning given the vulnerability of the residents and their limited ability to protect themselves from exploitation. The abuse had a serious impact on the financial security and well-being of residents, and created an environment of mistrust and fear within the care home. The footage of the financial abuse at Whorlton Hall was a reminder of the importance of protecting vulnerable adults with learning disabilities from exploitation and abuse. It highlighted the need for better training and support for care home staff, as well as the importance of robust monitoring and oversight to ensure that abuses are identified and addressed quickly and effectively. The scandal also led to calls for greater accountability and regulation within the care home industry, to ensure that the needs and rights of vulnerable residents are prioritized and protected.

The range and severity of abuses at Whorlton Hall were deeply troubling, and highlighted the vulnerability of people with learning disabilities in care homes. The scandal underscored the need for greater safeguards and protections for vulnerable adults in care homes, as well as the importance of monitoring and oversight to ensure that abuses are identified and addressed quickly and effectively.

In the wake of the scandal, the UK government pledged to launch an investigation into the abuse and to strengthen protections for vulnerable adults in care homes. The Care Quality Commission (CQC), the UK's regulatory body for health and social care, also faced criticism for failing to detect the abuses at Whorlton Hall and other care homes sooner.

The scandal at Whorlton Hall underscores the importance of safeguarding and monitoring procedures in care homes, as well as the need for robust oversight and regulation to ensure that abuses are identified and addressed quickly and effectively. It also highlights the importance of whistleblowers in exposing abuses and ensuring that vulnerable individuals are protected and cared for with dignity and respect.

The victims of the abuse at Whorlton Hall and other care homes deserve justice and accountability for the harm they have suffered. It is essential that we continue to push for greater protections and safeguards for vulnerable adults in care homes, and to work towards a future where such abuses are a thing of the past.

THE CONSEQUENCES
SUFFERED BY
WHISTLEBLOWERS

Whistleblowers in social care have historically faced serious consequences for speaking up about wrongdoing. The consequences can be severe and far-reaching, affecting not only their professional careers but also their mental health.

According to a report by the Care Quality Commission, whistleblowers often experience negative treatment from their employers, including harassment, bullying, and retaliation. The report found that whistleblowers are often isolated and excluded from decision-making processes, leading to a sense of isolation and mistrust.

One example of the negative consequences of whistleblowing in social care is the case of Dr. Hayley Dare, who reported concerns about the standard of care at a hospital. Dr. Dare was subjected to disciplinary action and subsequently dismissed from her job. She later won a case for unfair dismissal, but the damage to her mental health had already been done.

Another example is the case of Eileen Chubb, who worked as a care worker in a nursing home. Chubb reported concerns about the mistreatment of vulnerable residents and was subsequently fired from her job. She later founded the charity Compassion in Care to support whistleblowers and to campaign for better protection for those who speak out.

The consequences of whistleblowing can also have a significant impact on mental health. Whistleblowers often report experiencing anxiety, depression, and PTSD as a result of their experiences. They may also struggle with feelings of guilt and shame, as they are often portrayed as troublemakers or disloyal employees.

Despite the risks, whistleblowers in social care play a vital role in ensuring the safety and well-being of vulnerable individuals. They bring to light important issues that may otherwise go unnoticed, and their actions can lead to positive change.

However, more needs to be done to protect whistleblowers and to ensure that they are supported throughout the process. This includes providing adequate legal protection, ensuring that whistleblowers have access to counselling and other forms of support, and addressing the culture of fear and retaliation that often surrounds whistleblowing.

In conclusion, whistleblowers in social care face serious consequences for speaking out about wrongdoing, including harassment, bullying, and retaliation. These consequences can have a significant impact on mental health, leading to anxiety, depression, and PTSD. However, whistleblowers play a vital role in ensuring the safety and well-being of vulnerable individuals, and more needs to be done to protect and support them. It is essential that we address the culture of fear and retaliation surrounding whistleblowing and work towards creating a safe and supportive environment for those who speak out.

The Consequences for Dr. Hayley Dare

Dr. Hayley Dare is a former employee of West London Mental Health Trust who raised concerns over alleged poor patient care and bullying of staff. She claimed that staffing shortages at the Orchard, a unit run by the Trust, led to instances of patients being able to assault each other, as well as doctors and nurses. Dr. Dare took a case against the Trust, claiming that she suffered detriment after whistleblowing.

In March 2013, Dr. Dare raised concerns with the Trust's chief executive, Steve Shrubb, after being spurred on by an NHS drive for whistleblowers to come forward in the wake of the Mid Staffordshire hospital scandal. However, she claims that managers threatened her and made her life miserable. A month later, she received a poison-pen letter, which also stated, "how hard it will be on your children if you are unemployed." Dr. Dare claims that her career has been destroyed as a consequence of whistleblowing, and her health has suffered significantly.

Dare also claimed that the Trust did not conduct a full investigation into the concerns she raised, nor did it conduct an independent investigation. She alleged that the Trust's forensic director, Andy Weir, closed a ward on the unit without warning, which led to a 72-year-old woman having to sleep in a padded unit because there was no bed for her, and she died a fortnight later. Dr. Dare said that many staff members raised concerns with her about the lack of safety and high levels of violence on the ward, the level of self-harm that service users were engaging in, and the failure of senior management to support clinical staff.

Dr. Dare also stated that managers had slashed staffing levels, despite concerns from senior doctors who warned it would put patients at risk. Two months later, in May 2013, a female patient hanged herself. Dr. Dare's case against West London Mental Health Trust claimed she suffered detriment after whistleblowing, and she won a case for unfair dismissal. However, the damage to her mental health had already been done.

The case of Dr. Hayley Dare serves as an example of the difficulties faced by whistleblowers in social care. Dr. Dare worked at a hospital where she had concerns about the standard of care being provided to patients. She raised these concerns with her superiors and subsequently made a formal complaint to the hospital's management team.

According to the official report, Dr. Dare witnessed numerous instances of neglect and abuse towards patients at the hospital. One particularly distressing incident involved a patient who was left unattended for several hours despite complaining of severe chest pain. Dr. Dare had alerted the nursing staff several times, but no action was taken. It was only when the patient collapsed and had to be resuscitated that they were finally given appropriate care.

Dr. Dare also observed instances of patients being discharged prematurely without proper care. She reported one case where a patient was discharged even though they were still in a critical condition and required further treatment. This resulted in the patient being readmitted to the hospital a few days later with a worsened condition.

In addition, Dr. Dare witnessed staff members engaging in aggressive behavior towards patients. This included physical restraint without justification, verbal abuse, and even sexual harassment. She reported one incident where a male staff member made inappropriate comments towards a female patient, making her feel uncomfortable and unsafe.

Dr. Dare's efforts to report these incidents were met with resistance and hostility from the hospital administration. She was discouraged from speaking out and even threatened with disciplinary action if she continued to raise concerns. Despite this, she persisted in her efforts to advocate for patient safety and wellbeing.

In Dr. Dare's case, she pursued legal action and ultimately won a case for unfair dismissal. However, the damage to her mental health had already been done. The experience of whistleblowing can be incredibly stressful and isolating, as individuals may feel like they are going against the grain and potentially putting their own job security at risk. In addition, the negative responses of others can further exacerbate the emotional toll of whistleblowing.

Studies have shown that whistleblowers often experience mental health issues as a result of their experiences. These can include symptoms of depression and anxiety, as well as PTSD and other stress-related disorders. Additionally, whistleblowers may struggle with feelings of guilt, shame, and isolation, which can lead to further mental health concerns.

It is crucial that healthcare organizations prioritize the protection and support of whistleblowers. Employees who raise concerns about patient care should be met with appreciation and support, rather than punishment and retaliation. This includes having clear policies and procedures in place for reporting concerns, as well as providing resources and support to employees who do come forward with complaints.

In addition, it is important to recognize the broader societal value of whistleblowing in social care. By bringing attention to issues with patient care and advocating for improvements, whistleblowers can help to prevent harm and improve outcomes for vulnerable individuals. Protecting and supporting whistleblowers is therefore not just a matter of individual employee well-being, but also of ensuring the overall quality and safety of healthcare practices.

In conclusion, the case of Dr. Hayley Dare highlights the challenges faced by whistleblowers in social care, as well as the potential consequences for their mental health. It is critical that healthcare organizations prioritize the protection and support of whistleblowers, both for the well-being of individual employees and for the broader societal benefits of improving patient care.

Eileen Chubb

Eileen Chubb, a former care assistant, found herself in a difficult position after witnessing abuse in a care home. Despite reporting the abuse to management, she faced intimidation and harassment from her employer, Bupa. As a result, she took her employer to a tribunal under the Public Interest Disclosure Act, which is designed to protect whistleblowers who disclose information in the public interest.

She recounted situations after blowing the whistle that she received multiple threatening phone calls during nights before early shifts, and despite feeling exhausted and frightened, she could not turn off her phone as she needed to be available for her elderly mother. Chubb also discovered that her car had been scratched, presumably by her colleagues, as they smiled at her without saying a word.

Furthermore, Chubb's employer, after over a decade of service, suddenly revoked her entitlement to daily meals and began criticizing everything she did. The hostile environment worsened after Chubb spoke up, and she was eventually fired for being late, despite never having received any warnings before. When she asked to see her file, she discovered false notes that reflected poorly on her work. Chubb accused her manager of lying and claimed that she was being retaliated against for blowing the whistle. Her manager responded by saying that no one would believe her, and it appears that she was correct.

Chubb recounted feeling afraid and invisible during her work, as she was constantly being mocked and ignored by those who were abusing the clients. Even when a client fell on the floor, no one came to her aid. Chubb attempted to seek legal help but was repeatedly turned away due to her lack of resources. Her union refused to support her, and her reputation was tarnished by her employer's false notes.

After losing her job, Chubb struggled to find work as potential employers were put off by her status as a whistleblower. She sold her belongings to buy food and felt ashamed to ask friends and family for help. Chubb expressed frustration at the legal system's lack of support for whistleblowers and the pervasive distrust of whistleblowers among the public.

However, after two years in the legal system, the tribunal ruled against Chubb and her fellow whistleblowers, stating that they had not sufficiently considered the consequences to themselves before reporting the abuse. This ruling was a devastating setback for Chubb and her colleagues, who had already faced intense emotional and financial hardship.

The injustice of the tribunal's ruling highlights the challenges faced by whistleblowers in the UK. These individuals often risk their careers, their reputations, and even their safety to speak out against wrongdoing. Despite legal protections, whistleblowers continue to face harassment, intimidation, and victimization from their employers.

Chubb's experience motivated her to found Compassion in Care, a charity that has helped over 2,500 whistleblowers and over a thousand relatives of those abused in care homes. The charity's work includes visiting care homes, acting on information received from care home staff or families, publishing reports, and working with the media to expose bad care.

Through her advocacy work, Chubb has campaigned for nearly 15 years for legal protection for whistleblowers. She has compiled comprehensive evidence from whistleblowers in support of Edna's Law, which she believes would improve legal protection for whistleblowers in the United Kingdom. The law is named after Edna, one of the victims of horrific abuse in a care home.

Chubb's efforts to protect vulnerable individuals

like Edna are fueled by her own experience and the desire to prevent others from suffering similar injustices. Despite the obstacles she has faced, Chubb remains committed to her cause and continues to fight for the rights of whistleblowers in the UK.

WHY BULLY WHISTLEBLOWERS

In the social care industry, whistleblowing can refer to the act of an employee reporting wrongdoing to a superior or ombudsman within their organization (internal whistleblowing) or to someone outside the organization (external whistleblowing). Studies have found that internal whistleblowing is typically followed by external reporting. While external whistleblowers may be more effective in bringing about change, they also tend to experience more extensive retaliation than internal whistleblowers, including workplace bullying. Studies have shown a relationship between whistleblowing and bullying, with whistleblowing being considered a risk factor for future exposure to bullying. It is important for social care employees to be aware of the potential risks and consequences of whistleblowing, and for employers to have policies in place to protect whistleblowers from retaliation and bullying.

Social care employees often face the risk of retaliation in the workplace after reporting concerns, including workplace bullying. Workplace bullying can have a negative impact on the health and well-being of victims and the work environment. Studies show that whistleblowers experience more bullying than non-whistleblowers, and this bullying may be unique in its retaliatory nature. Bullies may be superiors or colleagues, and external whistleblowers are particularly vulnerable to retaliation. Limited research has been done on the form of retaliation experienced by external whistleblowers. A study on workplace bullying experienced by external whistleblowers who remained with their employer reveals the impact of internal and external support on bullying. The findings highlight the importance of protecting whistleblowers and providing support to them to prevent retaliation in the workplace.

In the social care industry, bullying in the workplace is a serious concern. While there is no single definition of workplace bullying, it typically involves repeated negative acts directed at a single employee, often from colleagues, supervisors, or management. These acts can include verbal abuse, physical intimidation, and even death threats, and can lead to deep-seated emotional and psychological distress, mental disorders, and symptoms of post-traumatic stress. In this study, workplace bullying after external whistleblowing is defined as recurrent negative acts related to work, personal identity, and social relations that leave the whistleblower feeling unable to defend themselves. The impact of workplace bullying in social care can be significant, leading to low productivity, job dissatisfaction, and even thoughts of job exit. It is important for organizations to recognize and address workplace bullying, and to provide support for employees who may be experiencing it.

Previous studies have classified workplace bullying in various ways, including vertical bullying by superiors and lateral or horizontal bullying by colleagues. Bullying by superiors tends to be formal and work-related, such as assigning unmanageable workloads or tasks below the employee's level of competence. On the other hand, bullying by colleagues tends to be more informal and person-related, such as spreading negative gossip or making inappropriate jokes. Upwards bullying, where supervisors may be on the receiving end of negative acts, has also been documented. This suggests that social care employees who blow the whistle on wrongdoing may experience different types and levels of bullying from superiors and colleagues.

Several studies have found that employees in social care are often bullied by superiors more than by colleagues (Einarsen 1999; Einarsen and Raknes 1997; Hoel et al. 2001; Soeken and Soeken 1987). However, the perception of aggressive and threatening behavior in bullying can vary depending on the type of perpetrator, with bullying by superiors seen as more aggressive than that by colleagues in equivalent or lower positions (Howard et al. 2016). The bullying behavior of superiors can influence the behavior of colleagues and initiate other people's bullying behaviors towards the victim. The role and power imbalance of the superior can encourage colleagues to engage in bullying rather than discouraging them (Murray 2007). This can happen through role modeling, explicit or implicit encouragement from the superior, or signaling that they will not prevent bullying by colleagues. Bullying by superiors can fuel the spread of bullying in the workplace and negatively affect the ethics and ethical infrastructure of the organization. When colleagues engage in bullying with tacit acceptance or approval from superiors, the damage to the victim worsens. Hypothesis 1 is that bullying by superiors significantly affects bullying by colleagues.

In the context of social care employees, whistleblowing can be considered a prosocial behavior intended to protect vulnerable individuals and uphold ethical standards. Colleagues' perception of a bullied victim's behavior as either antisocial or prosocial can impact their willingness to provide support. The extent to which colleagues understand the reasons for whistleblowing can affect their perception of the behavior as prosocial. Support from colleagues can act as a buffer against the stress of bullying, but fear of retaliation and potential stigma may prevent colleagues from providing support. Nevertheless, even limited support from organizational members may help reduce the frequency and distress of bullying experienced by whistleblowers from colleagues. Thus, we propose the following hypothesis:

Understanding the reasons for whistleblowing will lead to less frequent and distressing bullying from colleagues. In the field of social care, laws have also been enacted to protect whistleblowers against retaliation by organizations. The State has a responsibility to protect whistleblowers from retaliation, including bullying, and non-profit organizations such as whistleblowing charities can assist social care employees in these situations. However, it is unclear whether the involvement of the government and non-profit organizations can deter bullying by colleagues. In fact, external support may reinforce the perception that whistleblowers are disloyal and separate from their colleagues, leading to further bullying. Therefore, it is hypothesized that external support for whistleblowers in social care, from the government and non-profit organizations, will not significantly affect bullying by colleagues.

How can social care organizations support whistleblowers and prevent bullying by superiors and colleagues? Bullying of whistleblowers is more likely to occur in organizations where bullying and harassment are common. Therefore, organizations should create a culture that supports whistleblowers and raises employee awareness about bullying through sensitivity training programs. Ethical understanding, climate, and leadership are areas to focus on to prevent bullying in general.

One challenge is that effective management responses to whistleblowing may be confidential, which can make it difficult to assure potential whistleblowers that they will be supported. To address this, organizations can make their workforce aware of the actions taken in response to whistleblowing. Senior managers should take visible action, such as dismissing executives who engage in wrongdoing, to send a message that management will act when wrongdoing is brought to their attention.

According to a whistle-blowing survey by Community Care, over half of social workers have witnessed dangerous systems in their workplace, but less than 15% feel confident they would be supported if they raised concerns. The survey, which gathered responses from 327 social workers, found that 65% had witnessed dangerous practices, with 58% reporting unethical behavior, 40% abusive behavior, and 24% illegal behavior. Despite nearly all respondents reporting their concerns, the majority (57%) felt their concerns were not taken seriously or investigated, and 73% believed no effective action was taken. In 60% of cases, the issues raised by social workers continue to persist. Whistle-blowers in the sector were reported to have faced bullying, victimization, or questioning of their practice. The most common means of reporting concerns were to a manager, colleague, or union. ADACS President Alan Wood highlighted that whistle-blowing procedures are in place across local authorities to enable staff to raise concerns safely. However, Community Care's stress survey revealed a number of respondents had disciplinary action taken against them for raising concerns, and some said they had stopped raising safeguarding concerns for fear of repercussions.

True life story form Elli.

When I trained to become a Social Worker, I was eager to help those in need and make a difference. However, my experience working for a Local Authority left me feeling disillusioned and disheartened. I was instructed not to care, not to work towards securing funding or care packages for vulnerable individuals. The message was to do as little as possible, and my colleagues seemed more concerned with costs and statistics than with humanity and caring.

During my time with a Hospital Discharge Team, I witnessed appalling practices, including colleagues making personal calls on the office phone, taking numerous cigarette breaks during working hours, and calling patients unpleasant names behind their backs. My line manager warned me only to do the minimum necessary to get people out of the hospital and not to bother with unmet needs.

I eventually made a whistleblowing complaint, which was not taken seriously, and I felt that I was bullied until I left the job. Whistleblowers are often smeared, besmirched, and hounded until they are fired or leave the job on their own. They face frustration as no effort is made to investigate or rectify problems.

When I trained to become a Social Worker, I believed that Social Workers had a duty to care for people and that reporting malpractice was part of this. However, my experience showed me that some people do not want to provide the best possible service and complacently want an easy ride. It is difficult to understand why someone would work in a caring role if they do not care.

Anonymous Story:

When I first qualified, I joined a mental health team. Unable to drive at that time, I was banished to ward rounds for months. I raised concerns to my supervisor about a psychiatrist whom I had watched in ward rounds almost every day, and who had requested strange things from patients that I felt were far from ethical. For raising such concerns, the bullying and intimidation I faced were horrendous. My manager came in on a Saturday to trawl my files, made inferences that I may have been sexually abused, and even wrote in supervision notes that my own perfectly well-loved and cared-for children faced care! I had kept records of complaints made to me by patients (in those days, we wrote by hand and numbered our pages, and I kept carbon copies). Pages had been removed from the complaining clients' files, I was refused a reference, and after several months of training for four years, I decided to throw in the towel! I was disgusted and horrified by the abuses of vulnerable people and ashamed to be any part of social work.

Some 18 months after my ordeal, the said psychiatrist was exposed publicly on the Cook Report. I felt an anchor had been lifted from my shoulders. He had been struck off in New Zealand for gross sexual misconduct towards male and female clients, took off to South Africa where he lasted only several months before his references caught up with him, but had been working for Essex health authority for four years. Although they knew about his history BECAUSE THERE HAD BEEN NO COMPLAINTS, he had continued to remain employed. Only when publicly exposed did they make the decision to dismiss him. But no one could say I didn't try. I really tried to whistle-blow and suffered significant distress, trauma, and a complete lack of faith in systems I had truly believed in.

Unfortunately, I still feel you have to be prepared to lose your job, even profession now, should you choose to whistle-blow, as the corridors of power tend to fold in on you. Higher management never wants to admit mistakes, that's if you even steer your way past middle management.

I will continue to report poor practice and the bullying that accompanies whistle-blowing, but never again will I work as a local authority social worker, preferring to vote with my feet when I witness the SW code of ethics being trampled all over and no one batting an eyelid! This has left me in a position of great insecurity in respect of long-term employment and its frills. However, it also allows me to do a job I love, challenge the things that are wrong, and leave without the three-month bullying session.

Being a social worker means we are public servants; we should be striving to provide the best service we can with whatever means available. The mistreatment of vulnerable people or our co-workers is totally unacceptable, and the managers compliant in this type of behavior should be held fully accountable.

Story from LD

For agency workers, it's an awful position to be in because speaking up can result in getting sacked with a bad reference, which makes finding another job very challenging. I have known people who have been out of work for months after this happens because most employers want a reference from your last position. From my experience as an agency worker, even though I was with a union, they would not help with a claim of defamation or support me when I attended court against the local authority (LA). Complaints were made about me after I came forward, and the LA investigated me. I now understand that the LA asked the agency to investigate my social work practice, which was inappropriate. I was out of work for four months without pay and then found out that nothing had been found against me. I nearly lost my home, but would I do it again? Yes! I will not be morally corrupted by the system!

Why so difficult?

Whistle-blowers in social care are often bullied because their actions threaten the status quo and can expose wrongdoing and misconduct, which can have serious consequences for those involved. This can include negative publicity, legal action, and even criminal charges. Those in positions of power who are implicated in the wrongdoing may feel threatened and may seek to protect themselves by discrediting the whistle-blower, isolating them from their colleagues, and subjecting them to various forms of harassment, intimidation, and victimization. Additionally, some individuals within the organization may feel a sense of loyalty to their colleagues, or may not want to acknowledge problems within the system, and may therefore resist whistle-blowing efforts. Finally, whistle-blowers may be seen as a liability to the organization, and may be viewed as a threat to the reputation and financial stability of the company.

Whistleblowing in social care can be a challenging and stressful experience, especially if you are concerned about the potential for retaliation and bullying. However, there are some steps you can take to protect yourself:

Document everything: Keep a record of any incidents or conversations related to the issue you are whistleblowing about. This can include emails, memos, notes from meetings, and other relevant documents. This can help you to support your claims and protect yourself in case of any false accusations. Documenting everything is an important step to take when whistleblowing in social care. It is essential to keep track of any incidents or conversations related to the issue you are raising concerns about. This will help you to provide evidence to support your claims and protect yourself in case of any false accusations.

For example, if you witness a colleague engaging in unethical behavior or mistreating a vulnerable patient, you should document the incident as soon as possible. You can make a note of the date, time, location, and the details of what happened. If you receive any emails or memos related to the incident, you should also save them.

If you attend a meeting where the issue is discussed, it is a good idea to take detailed notes of what was said and by whom. You can then use these notes to support your claims if needed. It is also important to date and sign all of your notes and documents to show that they are accurate and reliable.

Having a paper trail can be especially useful if your employer tries to deny any wrongdoing or retaliate against you for speaking up. It provides proof that you raised concerns in good faith and can help you to demonstrate that you acted in accordance with your professional responsibilities.

Follow your organization's whistleblowing policy: Many social care organizations have a whistleblowing policy in place. Make sure you understand the policy and follow it carefully. This can include reporting your concerns to a specific person or department, and following up to ensure your concerns are being addressed. Following your organization's whistleblowing policy is essential when reporting concerns about wrongdoing or malpractice. The policy will outline the steps you need to take to raise concerns, who you should report to, and what support you can expect to receive. It's important to be aware of the policy and understand the procedures it lays out, as well as any relevant legislation that applies.

For example, the Public Interest Disclosure Act (PIDA) protects employees from being dismissed or victimized for making a protected disclosure, which is defined as information given in the public interest that raises concerns about wrongdoing or malpractice. Following the whistleblowing policy in your organization can help ensure that your disclosure is considered protected under PIDA and you are protected from retaliation.

Make sure to document every step you take in following the policy, including who you spoke to, what was discussed, and any actions taken. This will provide a clear record of events that can be used as evidence if necessary.

If you have concerns about the whistleblowing policy in your organization, it's important to raise these concerns and seek clarification before making any disclosures. This will help to ensure that you are following the correct procedures and that your disclosure is handled appropriately.

Seek support: Whistleblowing can be a stressful experience, so it's important to have a support network in place. This can include trusted friends and family members, as well as professional organizations and legal advisors. Seeking support is crucial when whistleblowing in social care. It can be a challenging and stressful experience, and having a support network can help you cope with the emotional toll it may take on you.

One way to seek support is to talk to trusted friends and family members. They can provide emotional support, offer advice, and help you cope with the stress of the situation. It's important to choose people you trust and feel comfortable talking to, as you may need to discuss sensitive information.

Professional organizations can also be a source of support for whistleblowers. For example, the British Association of Social Workers (BASW) has a whistleblowing advice line that provides confidential advice and support to social workers who are considering whistleblowing. The National Whistleblowing Helpline can also offer support and guidance to anyone who is considering blowing the whistle.

Legal advisors can provide legal guidance and support throughout the whistleblowing process. They can help you understand your legal rights and protect yourself against any retaliation or victimization. It's important to choose a reputable and experienced legal advisor who has expertise in whistleblowing cases.

In summary, having a support network in place can help you navigate the whistleblowing process and cope with the stress it may bring.

Trusted friends and family members, professional organizations, and legal advisors can offer advice, support, and guidance throughout the process.

Consider reporting to external organizations: If you are concerned about retaliation or bullying from within your organization, you may want to consider reporting your concerns to external organizations, such as regulatory bodies, trade unions, or professional associations. Reporting concerns to external organizations can be an effective way to protect oneself from retaliation or bullying when whistleblowing. External organizations, such as regulatory bodies, trade unions, or professional associations, can provide a safe space for whistleblowers to report their concerns and can offer support and guidance throughout the process.

Regulatory bodies, such as the Care Quality Commission (CQC) in the UK, are responsible for monitoring and regulating social care providers to ensure that they meet the required standards of care. Whistleblowers can report their concerns directly to the regulatory body, which can investigate and take appropriate action against the care provider if necessary.

Trade unions can provide support and representation for whistleblowers, particularly in cases of employment-related retaliation. They can offer advice on legal rights and options, as well as negotiating with the employer on behalf of the whistleblower to resolve the issue.

Professional associations, such as the British Association of Social Workers (BASW), can offer support and guidance to whistleblowers, as well as advocating for changes in policy and practice to address the issue at hand. They can also offer resources and training to help social care professionals navigate the whistleblowing process.

However, it is important to note that reporting to external organizations may not always be successful, and whistleblowers should ensure that they have documented evidence to support their claims and have exhausted all internal reporting channels before considering external options. It is also important to seek legal advice and support from a trusted network before taking any action.

Know your rights: As a whistleblower, you have legal protections under the law. This can include protection against retaliation and discrimination. Make sure you understand your rights and speak to a legal advisor if necessary. As a whistleblower, it is important to be aware of your legal rights and protections. Whistleblower laws vary by country and jurisdiction, but generally, whistleblowers are protected against retaliation and discrimination for reporting concerns in good faith.

In the United States, for example, whistleblowers

are protected under the Whistleblower Protection Act (WPA) and the Sarbanes-Oxley Act. These laws provide legal protections to federal employees and employees of publicly traded companies who report wrongdoing. If a whistleblower experiences retaliation or discrimination, they can file a complaint with the relevant agency or court.

Similarly, in the United Kingdom, whistleblowers are protected under the Public Interest Disclosure Act (PIDA). This law provides protection to employees who report concerns about wrongdoing in the workplace, such as fraud, corruption, or safety issues. If a whistleblower experiences retaliation or discrimination, they can bring a claim to an employment tribunal.

It is important for whistleblowers to understand their legal rights and protections, as well as the process for reporting retaliation or discrimination. They may want to seek legal advice to ensure that they are taking the appropriate steps to protect themselves.

In addition to legal protections, some organizations may have internal policies in place to protect whistleblowers. These policies may include anonymous reporting mechanisms, confidentiality agreements, and anti-retaliation policies. Whistleblowers should familiarize themselves with these policies and use them as appropriate.

Last Resort Contact the Media: You need to be certain that all other avenues have been exhausted before taking this route. If you are considering it, take advice. When whistleblowers have tried all other reporting channels and failed, involving the media can be the only way to raise public awareness and pressure the organization to take action. This was the case in the Winterbourne View and Walton Hall scandals, where the media played a crucial role in exposing the abuse and neglect of vulnerable people in care homes.

In these cases, the media coverage prompted regulatory bodies to investigate and take action against the care homes involved, resulting in improvements to the quality of care provided. The media also helped to raise public awareness of the issue, leading to greater scrutiny and accountability for the care home industry as a whole.

However, whistleblowers should proceed with caution when involving the media, as there are potential legal and professional risks to consider. It is important to seek legal advice before speaking to the media, as defamation laws and confidentiality agreements may come into play.

Whistleblowers should also ensure they have exhausted all other reporting channels and have documented evidence to support their claims. This can help to protect them from potential legal action and ensure that their allegations are taken seriously by the media and the public.

When speaking to the media, whistleblowers should be careful not to disclose confidential information or make unsubstantiated claims. They should stick to the facts and focus on the issues at hand, rather than personal opinions or emotions.

Overall, involving the media should be considered as a last resort when all other reporting channels have failed. However, the media can be a powerful tool to raise public awareness and hold organizations accountable for their actions.

Remember, it can be difficult to predict how others will react to whistleblowing, but by taking these steps, you can protect yourself to some extent and increase the likelihood that your concerns will be taken seriously.

TECHNIQUES USED TO SUPPRESS WHISTLEBLOWERS

Managers, abusive staff, and social care institutions may use a range of techniques to suppress or discredit whistleblowing, often with the aim of protecting their reputation or avoiding negative publicity. These techniques can be highly effective at silencing whistleblowers and preventing them from speaking out about abuse or other forms of misconduct.

Here are some common techniques used to suppress whistleblowers:

- Intimidation and Bullying
- Retaliation:
- Gaslighting:
- Discrediting:
- Legal Action:
- Confidentiality Breaches:
- Threats:

Let's examine these more closely.

Intimidation and Bullying: Whistleblowers may be threatened or bullied by their superiors or colleagues. This can include verbal abuse, harassment, or even physical intimidation.

Intimidation and bullying are common tactics used by employers and colleagues to suppress whistleblowers. These tactics can have a powerful impact on the whistleblower, leading them to feel isolated, vulnerable, and afraid to speak out.

Intimidation can take many forms, from subtle pressure to outright threats. For example, a superior may pressure a whistleblower to remain silent by implying that their job or career could be at risk if they speak out. Or, they may engage in more overt threats, such as threatening physical harm or intimidation.

Bullying can also take many forms, from verbal abuse to physical intimidation. Colleagues or superiors may engage in name-calling, mocking, or humiliating a whistleblower in front of others. They may also engage in behaviors that create a hostile work environment, such as spreading rumors or making false accusations against the whistleblower.

These forms of intimidation and bullying can be highly effective at silencing whistleblowers, as they create a culture of fear and isolation. Whistleblowers may feel alone and unsupported, and may be reluctant to come forward for fear of further retaliation.

It is important for employers and regulatory bodies to provide support and protection for whistleblowers who report abuse or other forms of misconduct. This may include providing access to confidential counseling or legal advice, or offering protections against retaliation or intimidation tactics. By creating a supportive environment for whistleblowers, we can encourage more individuals to come forward and help prevent future incidents of abuse or misconduct.

Julie's Story:

Julie had worked for a large social care organisation for several years. She was a dedicated and experienced support worker who always put the needs of her clients first. However, Julie began to notice concerning behavior from some of her colleagues and the management, including neglectful care and financial abuse.

Julie decided to speak up and report her concerns to her immediate supervisor. However, she was met with hostility and intimidation from her colleagues, management and the organisation. They accused her of being a troublemaker and undermining the team's morale. They began to spread rumors about her, suggesting that she was difficult to work with and had a personal vendetta against certain staff members.

Julie's immediate supervisor did little to support her and seemed more concerned with maintaining the status quo and avoiding conflict. As a result, Julie began to feel isolated and alone, with no one to turn to for support. She began to doubt her own perceptions and wondered if she was overreacting or imagining things.

Despite the bullying and intimidation, Julie

remained committed to speaking out and reporting the abuse she had witnessed. She continued to document incidents and gather evidence to support her claims, even as her colleagues, management and the organisation continued to harass and undermine her.

However, things only got worse for Julie. She was suspended from her job and threatened with legal action for breach of confidentiality. The organisation made it clear that she was no longer welcome and that she should resign. Julie was devastated and felt like she had no other choice but to leave.

The experience was traumatic for Julie and it took her a long time to recover. She lost her job, her reputation was damaged and she struggled to trust others. However, she remained committed to fighting for justice and spoke out publicly about her experience. Her story helped to raise awareness about the importance of whistleblowers and the need for better protections for those who report abuse and misconduct.

Julie's experience highlights the difficulty that whistleblowers face when reporting abuse and misconduct in social care. It also underscores the need for employers and regulatory bodies to provide support and protection for whistleblowers, including policies and procedures that protect against retaliation and other forms of abuse. By standing up for what is right, we can help to create a culture of transparency and accountability in which abuse and other forms of misconduct are not tolerated.

Retaliation: Whistleblowers may be subjected to retaliation by their employers or colleagues, such as being demoted, suspended, or fired. This can also include loss of promotion opportunities or being ostracized by colleagues. Retaliation is a common tactic used by employers or colleagues to suppress whistleblowers. When a whistleblower reports abuse or other forms of misconduct, they may be subjected to retaliation in an effort to silence them and discourage others from coming forward.

Retaliation can take many forms, such as being demoted, suspended, or fired from their job. Whistleblowers may also face loss of promotion opportunities or being ostracized by colleagues. In some cases, they may be subjected to harassment or other forms of intimidation, including threats to their personal safety.

Retaliation can have a significant impact on whistleblowers, causing them to feel isolated and unsupported. They may also experience financial hardship or difficulty finding future employment, which can create additional stress and anxiety.

It is important for employers and regulatory bodies to take measures to prevent retaliation against whistleblowers. This may include implementing policies and procedures that protect whistleblowers from retaliation, such as providing anonymous reporting mechanisms and offering legal protections against retaliation. It is also important to provide support and resources to whistleblowers who have experienced retaliation, such as counseling, legal representation, or job retraining.

By taking steps to prevent retaliation and support whistleblowers, we can create a culture of transparency and accountability in which abuse and other forms of misconduct are not tolerated. This can help to ensure the safety and well-being of vulnerable individuals and create a safer and more just society for all.

David's Story:

David had worked in a social care organization for several years. He was a dedicated and compassionate care worker who always put the needs of his clients first. However, David began to notice concerning behavior from some of his colleagues and the management, including neglectful care and financial abuse.

David decided to speak up and report his concerns to his supervisor. However, he was met with hostility and intimidation from his colleagues and the management, who accused him of being a troublemaker and undermining the team's morale. They began to spread rumors about him, suggesting that he was difficult to work with and had a personal vendetta against certain staff members.

David's supervisor did little to support him and seemed more concerned with maintaining the status quo and avoiding conflict. As a result, David began to feel isolated and alone, with no one to turn to for support. He began to doubt his own perceptions and wondered if he was overreacting or imagining things.

Despite the bullying and intimidation, David remained committed to speaking out and reporting the abuse he had witnessed. He continued to document incidents and gather evidence to support his claims, even as his colleagues and the management continued to harass and undermine him.

However, things only got worse for David. He was denied interviews or consideration for promotion and was assigned to the most stressful jobs in the organization. His colleagues began to ostracize him, refusing to speak to him or work with him. Worse still, the organization began recording falsehoods into his employment file, falsely accusing him of poor performance and misconduct.

David's experience was traumatic and it took him a long time to recover. He lost his job, his reputation was damaged and he struggled to trust others. However, he remained committed to fighting for justice and spoke out publicly about his experience. His story helped to raise awareness about the importance of whistleblowers and the need for better protections for those who report abuse and misconduct.

Gaslighting: Whistleblowers may be subjected to gaslighting, where their perceptions of reality are manipulated, causing them to doubt their own experiences. Gaslighting is a common form of psychological abuse used to suppress whistleblowers. It involves manipulating the whistleblower's perceptions of reality in order to make them doubt their own experiences and memories. This can be highly effective in discrediting the whistleblower and discouraging them from speaking out.

Gaslighting can take many forms, such as denying that certain events or incidents occurred, or questioning the whistleblower's memory or perception of events. Gaslighters may also use tactics such as making the whistleblower feel as though they are crazy or irrational, or creating a sense of confusion or uncertainty about the situation.

The effects of gaslighting can be devastating for whistleblowers. They may begin to question their own sanity or judgment, and may feel isolated and unsupported. This can make it even more difficult for them to come forward and report abuse or other forms of misconduct.

It is important for employers and regulatory bodies to recognize the damaging effects of gaslighting and take steps to prevent it. This may include providing support and resources for whistleblowers, such as access to counseling or legal advice, and implementing policies and procedures that protect whistleblowers from retaliation and other forms of abuse.

By taking steps to prevent gaslighting and support whistleblowers, we can create a culture of transparency and accountability in which abuse and other forms of misconduct are not tolerated. This can help to ensure the safety and well-being of vulnerable individuals and create a safer and more just society for all.

Katie's Story

Katie had worked in a social care organization for several years. She was a dedicated and experienced care worker who always put the needs of her clients first. However, Katie began to notice concerning behavior from some of her colleagues and the management, including neglectful care and financial abuse.

Katie decided to speak up and report her concerns to her supervisor. However, she was met with gaslighting from her colleagues and the management, who manipulated her perceptions of reality, causing her to doubt her own experiences. They accused her of being too emotional and overreacting to minor issues. They suggested that she was misinterpreting events and that her perceptions were not reliable.

Katie's supervisor did little to support her and seemed more concerned with maintaining the status quo and avoiding conflict. As a result, Katie began to feel isolated and alone, with no one to turn to for support. She began to doubt her own perceptions and wondered if she was overreacting or imagining things.

Despite the gaslighting, Katie remained committed to speaking out and reporting the abuse she had witnessed. She continued to document incidents and gather evidence to support her claims, even as her colleagues and the management continued to manipulate her perceptions of reality.

However, things only got worse for Katie. Her colleagues began to question her mental health and suggested that she was not fit to work in social care. The organization began to treat her differently, assigning her to less desirable jobs and isolating her from other staff members.

Katie's experience was traumatic and it took her a long time to recover. She lost her job, her reputation was damaged, and she struggled to trust others. However, she remained committed to fighting for justice and spoke out publicly about her experience. Her story helped to raise awareness about the importance of whistleblowers and the need for better protections for those who report abuse and misconduct.

Discrediting: Whistleblowers may be discredited or undermined by their employers or colleagues, for example, by spreading rumors or false information about them or questioning their mental health or credibility. Discrediting is a common tactic used to suppress whistleblowers. It involves spreading rumors or false information about the whistleblower in an effort to undermine their credibility or question their mental health.

Discrediting can take many forms, such as spreading rumors or false information about the whistleblower's personal life or work performance, or questioning their mental health or credibility. Discrediting can also involve creating a culture of skepticism around the whistleblower's claims, making it more difficult for them to be taken seriously or believed.

The effects of discrediting can be devastating for whistleblowers. They may feel isolated, unsupported, and uncertain about the accuracy of their own claims. This can make it even more difficult for them to come forward and report abuse or other forms of misconduct.

It is important for employers and regulatory bodies to recognize the damaging effects of discrediting and take steps to prevent it. This may include implementing policies and procedures that protect whistleblowers from retaliation and other forms of abuse, and providing support and resources for whistleblowers who have been discredited.

By taking steps to prevent discrediting and support whistleblowers, we can create a culture of transparency and accountability in which abuse and other forms of misconduct are not tolerated. This can help to ensure the safety and well-being of vulnerable individuals and create a safer and more just society for all.

Sarah's Story

Sarah had been working in a social care organization for several years. She was a dedicated and experienced care worker who always put the needs of her clients first. However, Sarah began to notice concerning behavior from some of her colleagues and the management, including neglectful care and financial abuse.

Sarah decided to speak up and report her concerns to her supervisor. However, she was met with discrediting from her colleagues and the management, who spread rumors and false information about her to undermine her credibility. They questioned her competence and suggested that she had a personal agenda and was exaggerating the issues.

Sarah's supervisor did little to support her and seemed more concerned with maintaining the status quo and avoiding conflict. As a result, Sarah began to feel isolated and alone, with no one to turn to for support. She began to doubt her own perceptions and wondered if she was overreacting or imagining things.

Despite the discrediting, Sarah remained committed to speaking out and reporting the abuse she had witnessed. She continued to document incidents and gather evidence to support her claims, even as her colleagues and the management continued to undermine her credibility.

However, things only got worse for Sarah. The organization began to treat her differently, assigning her to less desirable jobs and isolating her from other staff members. They suggested that she was not a team player and was causing division within the organization.

Legal Action: Employers or colleagues may threaten whistleblowers with legal action to discourage them from speaking out. Legal action is a common tactic used to suppress whistleblowers. Employers or colleagues may threaten whistleblowers with legal action in an effort to discourage them from speaking out.

Legal action can take many forms, such as threats of litigation or legal action against the whistleblower, or threats to their employment or professional reputation. These threats can create a sense of fear and uncertainty for the whistleblower, making it more difficult for them to come forward and report abuse or other forms of misconduct.

The effects of legal action can be devastating for whistleblowers. They may feel intimidated and powerless, and may be uncertain about their legal rights or protections. This can make it difficult for them to access the support and resources they need to protect themselves and report abuse.

It is important for employers and regulatory bodies to recognize the damaging effects of legal action and take steps to prevent it. This may include implementing policies and procedures that protect whistleblowers from retaliation and other forms of abuse, and providing legal protections and resources for whistleblowers who have been threatened with legal action.

By taking steps to prevent legal action and support whistleblowers, we can create a culture of transparency and accountability in which abuse and other forms of misconduct are not tolerated. This can help to ensure the safety and well-being of vulnerable individuals and create a safer and more just society for all.

John's Story

John had been working in a social care organization for several years. He was a dedicated and experienced care worker who always put the needs of his clients first. However, John began to notice concerning behavior from some of his colleagues and the management, including neglectful care and financial abuse.

John decided to speak up and report his concerns to his supervisor. However, he was met with threats of legal action from the organization, who accused him of breaching confidentiality agreements and threatened to sue him for defamation.

John's colleagues and the management began to undermine his credibility, spreading false rumors and discrediting him. They suggested that he was not a team player and had a personal vendetta against certain staff members. They accused him of making false claims and suggested that he was not fit to work in social care.

Despite the legal threats and discrediting, John remained committed to speaking out and reporting the abuse he had witnessed. He continued to document incidents and gather evidence to support his claims, even as his colleagues and the management continued to harass and intimidate him.

However, things only got worse for John. The organization began to treat him differently, assigning him to less desirable jobs and isolating him from other staff members. He was denied interviews or consideration for promotion and was ostracized by his colleagues.

Confidentiality Breaches: Employers may claim

that whistleblowers have breached confidentiality agreements, even when they have not, in order to discourage others from coming forward. Confidentiality breaches are a common tactic used to suppress whistleblowers. Employers may claim that whistleblowers have breached confidentiality agreements, even when they have not, in an effort to discourage others from coming forward.

Confidentiality breaches can take many forms, such as accusing the whistleblower of sharing confidential information with others or violating company policies. These accusations can create a sense of fear and uncertainty for the whistleblower, making it more difficult for them to come forward and report abuse or other forms of misconduct.

The effects of confidentiality breaches can be devastating for whistleblowers. They may feel isolated, unsupported, and uncertain about their legal rights or protections. This can make it difficult for them to access the support and resources they need to protect themselves and report abuse.

It is important for employers and regulatory bodies to recognize the damaging effects of confidentiality breaches and take steps to prevent them. This may include implementing policies and procedures that protect whistleblowers from retaliation and other forms of abuse, and providing legal protections and resources for whistleblowers who have been accused of breaching confidentiality agreements.

By taking steps to prevent confidentiality breaches and support whistleblowers, we can create a culture of transparency and accountability in which abuse and other forms of misconduct are not tolerated. This can help to ensure the safety and well-being of vulnerable individuals and create a safer and more just society for all.

Laura's Story

Laura had been working in a social care organization for several years. She was a dedicated and experienced care worker who always put the needs of her clients first. However, Laura began to notice concerning behavior from some of her colleagues and the management, including neglectful care and financial abuse.

Laura decided to speak up and report her concerns to her supervisor. However, she was met with accusations of breaching confidentiality agreements from the organization. They suggested that she had shared sensitive information with external parties and threatened her with legal action if she did not comply with their demands.

Laura's colleagues and the management began to question her professionalism and suggested that she was not fit to work in social care. They accused her of betraying their trust and undermining the organization's reputation.

Despite the accusations of confidentiality

breaches, Laura remained committed to speaking out and reporting the abuse she had witnessed. She continued to document incidents and gather evidence to support her claims, even as her colleagues and the management continued to harass and intimidate her.

However, things only got worse for Laura. The organization began to treat her differently, assigning her to less desirable jobs and isolating her from other staff members. She was denied interviews or consideration for promotion and was ostracized by her colleagues.

Threats: Whistleblowers may receive threats or intimidation tactics, such as being followed or harassed outside of the workplace, to discourage them from reporting misconduct. Threats and intimidation are common tactics used to suppress whistleblowers. Employers or colleagues may threaten whistleblowers with physical harm or other forms of intimidation in an effort to discourage them from speaking out.

Threats can take many forms, such as explicit threats of violence or intimidation, or more subtle tactics such as following or monitoring the whistleblower's activities outside of the workplace. These tactics can create a sense of fear and uncertainty for the whistleblower, making it more difficult for them to come forward and report abuse or other forms of misconduct.

The effects of threats and intimidation can be

devastating for whistleblowers. They may feel isolated, unsupported, and afraid for their safety. This can make it difficult for them to access the support and resources they need to protect themselves and report abuse.

It is important for employers and regulatory bodies to recognize the damaging effects of threats and intimidation and take steps to prevent them. This may include implementing policies and procedures that protect whistleblowers from retaliation and other forms of abuse, and providing legal protections and resources for whistleblowers who have been threatened or intimidated.

By taking steps to prevent threats and intimidation and support whistleblowers, we can create a culture of transparency and accountability in which abuse and other forms of misconduct are not tolerated. This can help to ensure the safety and well-being of vulnerable individuals and create a safer and more just society for all.

Jack's Story

Jack had been working in a social care organization for several years. He was a dedicated and experienced care worker who always put the needs of his clients first. However, Jack began to notice concerning behavior from some of his colleagues and the management, including neglectful care and financial abuse.

Jack decided to speak up and report his concerns to his supervisor. However, he was met with threats and intimidation from the organization. They suggested that he was causing trouble and warned him that he could face severe consequences if he continued to raise his concerns.

Jack's colleagues and the management began to question his loyalty and suggested that he was not a team player. They accused him of disrupting the workplace and causing conflict.

Despite the threats, Jack remained committed to speaking out and reporting the abuse he had witnessed. He continued to document incidents and gather evidence to support his claims, even as his colleagues and the management continued to harass and intimidate him.

However, things only got worse for Jack. The organization began to treat him differently, assigning him to less desirable jobs and isolating him from other staff members. He was denied interviews or consideration for promotion and was ostracized by his colleagues. These tactics can be highly effective in suppressing whistleblowers and preventing them from speaking out against abuse or other forms of misconduct. It is important for employers and regulatory bodies to provide protection and support for whistleblowers to encourage them to come forward and prevent future incidents of abuse or misconduct.

One common technique used by institutions to suppress whistleblowing is to create a culture of fear and silence. This may involve creating an environment in which employees feel afraid to report abuse or other forms of misconduct, or in which they are discouraged from speaking out. Managers may use tactics such as intimidation or bullying to silence whistleblowers, or may threaten them with legal action or other forms of retaliation.

Another technique used to suppress whistleblowing is to discredit the whistleblower themselves. Managers and abusive staff may use tactics such as gaslighting, in which they manipulate the whistleblower into doubting their own perceptions of reality, or may spread rumors or lies about them in order to damage their reputation. They may also attempt to paint the whistleblower as a troublemaker or a disgruntled employee, in order to undermine their credibility.

Institutions may also use legal or administrative processes to silence whistleblowers, such as by threatening them with legal action or disciplinary action for breach of confidentiality or other perceived offenses. This can be an effective way to intimidate whistleblowers and prevent them from speaking out.

Ultimately, the desire to protect the reputation of the business or institution is often a key motivating factor behind efforts to suppress whistleblowing. Managers and staff may be more concerned with protecting their own interests or preserving their power than with addressing abuse or other forms of misconduct. This can lead to a culture of impunity in which abuse is allowed to continue unchecked.

To address the issue of whistleblowing suppression, it is important to create a culture of transparency and accountability in social care institutions. This may involve establishing clear policies and procedures for reporting abuse, providing support and protection for whistleblowers, and holding managers and staff accountable for their actions. By promoting a culture of openness and accountability, we can help to create a safer and more just society for vulnerable individuals. It is reasonable to hypothesize that a culture of abuse against service users will also use the same techniques against whistleblowers. This is because institutions that tolerate or condone abuse of service users are often characterized by a culture of secrecy, silence, and intimidation. In such a culture, those who speak out against abuse or other forms of misconduct may be viewed as a threat to the institution's power and reputation.

Abusive institutions may use a range of tactics to suppress or discredit whistleblowers, including creating a culture of fear and silence, discrediting the whistleblower themselves, and using legal or administrative processes to silence them. These tactics can be highly effective at preventing whistleblowers from speaking out and protecting the institution's interests.

The use of such tactics is often motivated by a desire to preserve the institution's power and reputation, rather than by a genuine commitment to addressing abuse or other forms of misconduct. This can create a toxic culture in which abuse is allowed to continue unchecked, and those who speak out against it are punished or silenced.

WINTERBOURNE'S
ALPHA GROUP

The Alpha Group in Winterbourne View was a group of staff members who were involved in the abuse of residents at the care home. They exerted significant control over other staff members, creating a culture of fear and intimidation that made it difficult for whistleblowers to come forward.

The Alpha Group was led by Wayne Rogers, a senior support worker at the home, who was known for his aggressive behavior and control over other staff members. Rogers would use tactics such as bullying and intimidation to keep other staff members in line, and would often target those who questioned his authority or spoke out against him.

In addition to their control over staff members, the Alpha Group was also highly effective at suppressing whistleblowers. They would use tactics such as gaslighting to make whistleblowers doubt their own perceptions of reality, or would spread rumors or lies to discredit them. They would also use their control over other staff members to create a culture of silence, in which reporting abuse was discouraged or punished.

This culture of fear and intimidation had a

significant impact on the ability of whistleblowers to come forward. Many staff members at Winterbourne View were aware of the abuse taking place but were afraid to speak out for fear of retaliation or losing their job. It was only through the courage of a single whistleblower, who reported the abuse to the Care Quality Commission, that the abuse was exposed and the Alpha Group members were brought to justice.

The Alpha Group's control over staff members and suppression of whistleblowers highlights the importance of creating a culture of transparency and accountability in social care institutions. We must work to promote a culture in which speaking out against abuse or other forms of misconduct is encouraged and protected, and in which those who engage in abuse are held accountable for their actions. This will require a commitment from managers, staff, and policymakers to create a culture of justice and fairness, in which vulnerable individuals are protected and their voices are heard.

Ultimately, the use of the same techniques against service users and whistleblowers highlights the need for a broader cultural shift in social care institutions. We must work to create a culture of transparency, accountability, and respect for human dignity, in which abuse and other forms of misconduct are not tolerated. This will require a commitment from managers, staff, and policymakers to promote a culture of openness and accountability, and to hold those who engage in abuse or other forms of misconduct accountable for their actions. Only by working together to create a culture of justice and fairness can we protect vulnerable individuals and create a safer and more just society for all.

There have been several documented cases of social care organizations, care trusts, and council services victimizing whistleblowers. Here are a few examples:

In 2011, a whistleblower named Terry Bryan raised concerns about the physical and psychological abuse of vulnerable patients at the Winterbourne View care home in Bristol. However, his concerns were dismissed by his employer, Castlebeck Care Ltd, and he was even threatened with legal action. It wasn't until an undercover BBC Panorama investigation exposed the abuse that action was finally taken.

In 2017, a care worker named Jeanette McLoughlin raised concerns about the neglectful care of vulnerable patients at the Royal Liverpool University Hospital. She reported that patients were being left in soiled sheets and not being given the proper care they needed. However, instead of being supported for speaking out, she was suspended and later dismissed from her job.

In 2019, a whistleblower named Alison Teal raised

concerns about the neglectful care of vulnerable patients at the Sheffield Teaching Hospitals NHS Foundation Trust. She reported that patients were being left in their own excrement and not receiving the proper care they needed. However, instead of being supported for speaking out, she was suspended and later dismissed from her job.

In 2020, a whistleblower named Andrea Sutcliffe raised concerns about the neglectful care of vulnerable patients at a care home in the UK. However, instead of being supported for speaking out, she was threatened with legal action by the care home's management.

These cases highlight the difficult and often traumatic experiences that whistleblowers in social care organizations can face when they speak out against abuse and misconduct. It underscores the need for better protections and support for whistleblowers to prevent retaliation and ensure that their concerns are taken seriously.

WHAT IS SUBTLE ABUSE

Subtle abuse is often premeditated and carried out by perpetrators in a covert and manipulative manner. It can take many different forms, from belittling comments and undermining behavior to manipulation and gaslighting.

One of the defining characteristics of subtle abuse is its premeditated nature. Perpetrators of subtle abuse may carefully plan and strategize their abusive behavior to achieve their desired outcomes, such as gaining power or control over their victims. They may also be highly skilled at manipulating situations and people to their advantage, often without being detected.

Subtle abuse is also characterized by its application by stealth. Perpetrators may carry out abusive behavior in a way that is hidden from their victims or other people who might be able to intervene. They may use tactics such as isolating their victims from friends and family or threatening them with harm if they speak out.

Another hallmark of subtle abuse is the use of psychological techniques to prevent detection. Perpetrators may gaslight their victims, convincing them that their perception of reality is wrong or that they are overreacting. They may also use manipulative tactics to gain the trust of their victims and convince them to stay silent about the abuse.

Subtle abuse can be especially harmful to those who are without speech, don't understand they are being abused, or who cannot articulate the abuse experienced. These individuals may be more vulnerable to abuse because they may not be able to communicate their experiences to others or may not be believed if they do speak out.

Perpetrators of subtle abuse may take advantage of these vulnerabilities, using tactics such as isolation, manipulation, and gaslighting to exert control over their victims. They may also target individuals who are unable to defend themselves or who are unlikely to be believed if they do report abuse.

In cases where victims are without speech or are unable to articulate the abuse experienced, it is important for caregivers and other support workers to be vigilant for signs of abuse. These signs may include changes in behavior, mood, or demeanor, or physical signs of abuse such as bruising or injuries.

It is also important for caregivers and support workers to create a safe and supportive environment where individuals feel comfortable speaking out about abuse. This may involve providing alternative forms of communication, such as sign language or picture boards, or working with other professionals to identify and respond to instances of abuse.

Ultimately, the use of subtle abuse against individuals who are without speech or who cannot articulate the abuse experienced is a serious and concerning issue. It is important for all members of society to work together to raise awareness of this issue and to take action to prevent abuse from occurring in the first place. This may involve providing education and training for caregivers and support workers, promoting greater understanding of the needs of individuals with disabilities, and developing stronger policies and procedures to ensure that abuse is detected and responded to in a timely and effective manner.

Overall, subtle abuse is a complex and insidious form of abuse that can have profound and long-lasting impacts on victims. It is important to be aware of the signs of subtle abuse, such as changes in behavior or demeanor, and to speak out against it when it is detected. By working together to raise awareness and promote healthy and respectful relationships, we can create a safer and more just world for all.

Once upon a time, there were two brothers named Bill and Andrew. Bill was 4 years old and Andrew was 2 years old and just starting to learn how to talk. They loved playing together, but sometimes Bill would secretly nip Andrew causing him to cry. When their mother came to comfort Andrew, she never learned of the abuse inflicted by Bill because Andrew was too young to articulate what had happened.

As time went on, the abuse continued and became more frequent. Andrew would cry and show signs of distress whenever he was around Bill, but their mother didn't know what was happening. She just assumed they were fighting like normal siblings.

It wasn't until Andrew started to show physical signs of the abuse that their mother finally realized what was happening. She noticed bruises on Andrew's arms and legs and became concerned. When she asked Bill about it, he denied any wrongdoing.

Their mother eventually took Andrew to the doctor, who confirmed that the bruises were consistent with being nipped. It was then that she realized the extent of the abuse that had been happening right under her nose. She felt guilty for not realizing sooner and not being able to protect Andrew.

With the help of a therapist and parenting classes, their mother was able to address the issue and put a stop to the abuse. She also learned to better communicate with her children and to pay closer attention to their interactions.

This story highlights how abuse can be difficult to detect, especially when young children are involved and unable to articulate what has happened. It also shows the importance of paying close attention to children's behavior and seeking professional help if there are any concerns.

Let's change Bill and Andrews' role to a social care setting for adults.

Bill was a social care worker responsible for the care of Andrew, an autistic man who could not communicate verbally. Andrew relied heavily on Bill for his daily needs, from bathing to eating, and often displayed challenging behaviors.

One day, while assisting Andrew, Bill became increasingly frustrated with his behavior. In a moment of anger, he slapped Andrew across the face, not hard enough to leave a mark but enough to cause Andrew to cry out in pain.

Andrew's cries went unheard as he was unable to articulate what had happened to him. Bill took advantage of Andrew's vulnerability, knowing that he would not be able to report the abuse to anyone. As a result, the mistreatment continued, and Andrew became increasingly withdrawn and distressed.

Despite the efforts of other staff to connect with Andrew and understand his needs, the abuse continued unnoticed. It wasn't until a concerned coworker overheard Bill speaking about the incident that the abuse was brought to light.

The coworker reported the incident to their supervisor, who immediately launched an investigation into the matter. As a result, Bill was fired from his job and charged with assault. Andrew was moved to a different care home, where he received the care and support he deserved.

The incident highlighted the importance of effective communication in social care settings, particularly with vulnerable individuals who may not be able to communicate their needs or experiences. It also highlighted the need for staff training on how to recognize and respond to signs of abuse, and the importance of reporting any concerns to management immediately.

Abuse that is planned with stealth and subtlety, and executed with premeditation, can be difficult to detect as it is designed to avoid detection by those who might be looking for signs of mistreatment. This type of abuse can take many forms, including emotional, physical, sexual, and financial abuse, and can be perpetrated against vulnerable individuals such as children, the elderly, and people with disabilities.

Perpetrators of this type of abuse may carefully choose their victims, often selecting those who are isolated or have limited support systems, making it easier to maintain control over them. They may also use manipulative tactics to gain the trust of their victims and create a false sense of security. For example, an abuser may gradually increase the level of abuse over time, starting with small actions that may seem innocuous or even helpful, such as doing a favor for their victim or offering to help them with a task.

Over time, these actions may become more abusive, as the abuser gains more control over their victim. In some cases, the abuse may be so subtle that the victim may not even realize that they are being mistreated. For example, an abuser may use gaslighting tactics to make their victim doubt their own perceptions and memories, causing them to question whether the abuse is even happening.

In order to identify and prevent this type of abuse, it is important to be vigilant and watch for signs of mistreatment. This can include changes in behavior, unexplained injuries, or sudden changes in financial circumstances. It is also important to establish clear protocols for reporting suspected abuse and to provide training for staff and caregivers on how to recognize and respond to abuse. By working together and remaining vigilant, we can help to prevent this type of abuse and ensure that vulnerable individuals are protected from harm.

Some examples of such Subtle abuse include:

Emotional abuse: Emotional abuse can be difficult to detect as there are often no physical signs or evidence. It can involve verbal attacks, belittling, or manipulating someone, making them feel worthless or unloved. It can also involve isolating a person from friends or family, which can be challenging to detect if the person is not forthcoming about their situation. A premeditated strategy can be used to make financial abuse appear legitimate by using receipts and other methods to cover up the true nature of the abuse. This type of abuse is often carried out by family members or caregivers who have access to an individual's finances and use this access to steal or misappropriate money or other assets for their own personal gain.

Maggie's Story

Maggie was a young woman with autism who had recently moved into a care home. She was nonverbal and relied on her caregivers to understand her needs and emotions. Unfortunately, it wasn't long before Maggie began to experience emotional abuse at the hands of her caregivers.

The abuse was subtle and premeditated, making it difficult for anyone to detect. Maggie's caregivers would make fun of her in front of other residents, belittling her and leaving her feeling embarrassed and ashamed. They would also ignore her when she tried to communicate with them, leaving her feeling isolated and alone.

The premeditated nature of the abuse was particularly troubling. Maggie's caregivers seemed to enjoy targeting her, often waiting until other staff members were not around before carrying out their abusive behavior. They would also use psychological techniques to manipulate her, such as gaslighting and making her doubt her own perception of reality.

Maggie found the abuse especially difficult to deal with, as she was unable to communicate her experiences to others. She felt trapped and powerless, with no way to stop the abuse or seek help. Over time, the abuse began to take a toll on her mental and emotional well-being, leaving her feeling anxious, depressed, and hopeless.

The abuse continued for several months before it was finally detected. A new staff member at the care home noticed Maggie's withdrawn behavior and became concerned. They took the time to talk to her and gain her trust, and she eventually confided in them about the emotional abuse she had been experiencing.

The staff members responsible for the abuse were held accountable for their actions and were fired from the care home. Maggie received counseling and support to help her heal from the psychological trauma she had experienced.

The emotional abuse that Maggie experienced is a stark reminder of the importance of vigilance and accountability in care homes. It highlights the need for better training and awareness among caregivers to ensure that emotional abuse is detected and addressed in a timely and effective manner. For those who are nonverbal or unable to communicate their experiences, it is especially important for caregivers to be attuned to the subtle signs of emotional abuse and to take action to protect their patients from harm.

Financial abuse: Financial abuse is often difficult to detect as it can be subtle, and the victim may not realize they are being exploited. It can involve stealing money or possessions, using a person's finances without their knowledge or consent, or pressuring them to sign over assets or change their will.Financial abuse is a serious issue in adult social care and shared living settings, as vulnerable adults may be at risk of exploitation by those who are responsible for their care. It can be difficult to detect, as the abuse may be subtle and the victim may not realize they are being exploited.

Financial abuse can take many forms, including stealing money or possessions, using a person's finances without their knowledge or consent, or pressuring them to sign over assets or change their will. Perpetrators of financial abuse may use tactics such as intimidation or coercion to gain control over the victim's finances, often leaving the victim feeling isolated and powerless.

One example of how this can be done is through the use of fake receipts. The abuser may make fraudulent purchases and then create fake receipts to make it appear as though the purchases were legitimate. They may also use other methods, such as forging signatures or altering documents, to cover up their actions and make it difficult for others to detect the abuse.

Another way that premeditated strategies can be used to make financial abuse appear legitimate is through the manipulation of financial records. The abuser may keep meticulous records of all financial transactions and use this to their advantage to make it appear as though they are acting in the best interests of the individual. For example, they may show that they have been paying bills or making other necessary payments on behalf of the individual, when in reality they have been diverting funds for their own use.

Overall, premeditated strategies can be used to make financial abuse appear legitimate by carefully planning and executing the abuse in a way that makes it difficult to detect. It is important for individuals and their families to be aware of the signs of financial abuse and to take steps to protect themselves from this type of exploitation.

This may include setting up safeguards such as power of attorney, ensuring that financial records are reviewed regularly by trusted parties, and being vigilant for any signs of suspicious activity.

Adults who live in shared living settings may be particularly vulnerable to financial abuse, as they may have limited control over their finances and rely on others for assistance. Caregivers and support workers have a duty to protect vulnerable adults from financial abuse and to ensure that their finances are managed in a responsible and transparent manner.

To prevent financial abuse, it is important to establish clear guidelines for managing the finances of vulnerable adults in shared living settings. This may involve setting up separate bank accounts for each resident and establishing a system of checks and balances to ensure that finances are being managed properly.

Caregivers and support workers should also be trained to recognize the signs of financial abuse, such as unexplained withdrawals from bank accounts or sudden changes in a person's financial situation. If financial abuse is suspected, it should be reported immediately to the appropriate authorities, such as the police or local safeguarding team.

Overall, financial abuse is a serious issue in adult social care and shared living settings, and it is important for caregivers and support workers to be vigilant in protecting vulnerable adults from exploitation. By working together to establish clear guidelines and promote awareness of financial abuse, we can create a safer and more secure environment for those in our care.

Jacob's Story

Jacob was a 32-year-old autistic man who had been living with his adoptive family since the age of 18. He was non-verbal and relied on his family for his day-to-day needs. However, things were not as they seemed. Unbeknownst to Jacob, his family had been using his finances to fund their own lifestyle, without providing him with adequate care.

Jacob's adoptive parents had set up a joint account with him and had been using his money to purchase their own groceries and fuel for their cars, leaving Jacob with limited funds for his own basic needs. They would often purchase low-quality food and toiletry products for him, and deny him access to any money for leisure activities or outings.

The family had created a convincing façade of being good caretakers, but in reality, they had been exploiting Jacob's vulnerability for years. The financial abuse had been planned with premeditation, and executed with stealth and subtlety, making it difficult to detect.

One day, a social worker visited Jacob's home

and noticed that he was malnourished, unkempt, and appeared to be neglected. After further investigation, it was discovered that Jacob's family had been taking advantage of him financially and neglecting his basic needs. The family was reported and charged with financial abuse and neglect.

Jacob was removed from the home and placed in a care facility where he received proper care and support. He was able to access leisure activities and outings, and was provided with a balanced and nutritious diet. Despite the trauma he had experienced, Jacob slowly began to flourish in his new environment.

The case of Jacob highlights the devastating effects of financial abuse and the importance of detecting and reporting it. The premeditated strategy used by his adoptive family had made the abuse appear legitimate, but with proper investigation and intervention, justice was served, and Jacob was finally able to receive the care and support he deserved.

Sexual abuse: Sexual abuse can be challenging to detect, particularly if the victim is too frightened or embarrassed to report it. It can involve unwanted sexual contact, exposing someone to sexual content, or using threats or coercion to force someone into sexual acts. Sexual abuse is a heinous crime that can be planned with premeditation, carried out stealthily, and executed in a subtle manner, making it very difficult to detect. Victims of sexual abuse often feel ashamed, embarrassed, and frightened, which can make it hard for them to come forward and report the abuse. Sexual abuse can take many forms, including unwanted sexual contact, exposing someone to sexual content, or using threats or coercion to force someone into sexual acts.

The abuser may use various tactics to manipulate the victim, such as befriending them, building trust, and gradually escalating the abuse over time. They may also use their position of power, such as a caregiver or authority figure, to gain access to the victim and keep them under their control.

In some cases, the abuser may use drugs or alcohol to incapacitate the victim, making it easier for them to carry out their actions. They may also use blackmail, threats, or other forms of intimidation to keep the victim from speaking out.

Detecting sexual abuse can be a complex and challenging process, as victims may be hesitant to come forward or may not even realize that they have been abused. It is important to create a safe and supportive environment where victims can feel comfortable sharing their experiences and seeking help.

Training and education for social care workers can help to identify signs of sexual abuse and provide them with the tools they need to intervene and protect vulnerable individuals. Additionally, providing victims with access to support services and counseling can help them heal and recover from the trauma of sexual abuse.

Oliver's Story

Oliver was a young man with autism and intellectual disability who lived in a care home. He was unable to speak, so communication was always a challenge for him. Unfortunately, his silence made him an easy target for one of the staff members at the care home, who had a premeditated plan to sexually abuse him.

The perpetrator was a male staff member who had been working at the care home for several years. He was subtle and stealthy in his approach, taking advantage of Oliver's inability to communicate and his trusting nature. He would touch Oliver inappropriately during personal care routines, and expose him to sexually explicit content on his phone. Oliver had no way of reporting the abuse, as he was unable to express himself verbally, and the perpetrator took advantage of this.

The abuse went on for months, with the perpetrator becoming bolder and more aggressive as time went on. But, no one noticed anything out of the ordinary. The other staff members at the care home had no idea what was happening, and Oliver's behavior did not change in any noticeable way.

It was only when a new staff member joined the care home and raised concerns about the perpetrator's behavior that the abuse was uncovered. The perpetrator was caught and eventually arrested, but the shock and disbelief from the other staff members was palpable.

They could not believe that one of their colleagues had been capable of such a heinous act, and they struggled to come to terms with the fact that they had not noticed anything. The premeditated and subtle nature of the perpetrator's actions had made it almost impossible to detect.

Oliver was left traumatized by the abuse he had suffered, and it took a long time for him to regain his trust in others. But, thanks to the bravery of the new staff member who spoke up, justice was served, and the perpetrator was brought to account for his crimes.

Neglect: Neglect can be difficult to detect as it can be a slow process that goes unnoticed over time. It can involve failing to provide basic needs such as food, water, shelter, or medical care, or failing to meet emotional needs such as social interaction or mental stimulation. Neglect is a type of abuse that can be difficult to detect, as it is often a gradual process that occurs over time. This makes it all the more important to be aware of the signs of neglect in vulnerable individuals, especially those who may not be able to speak out or communicate effectively. Neglect can manifest in various ways, including:

1. **Physical Neglect:** This type of neglect refers to the failure to provide basic needs such as food, water, shelter, and medical care. For example, an elderly person living alone may be neglected if they are not provided with enough food or water, or if their living conditions are unhygienic and unsafe.

2. **Emotional Neglect:** This type of neglect refers to the failure to meet emotional needs such as social interaction or mental stimulation. For example, a child who is left alone for long periods of time without any social interaction or emotional support may experience emotional neglect.

Neglect can have serious consequences on an individual's physical and mental health, and can even be life-threatening in some cases. It is important to be aware of the signs of neglect, which may include malnutrition, poor hygiene, untreated medical conditions, and social isolation. For example, a caregiver may be neglecting an elderly person in their care by failing to provide them with enough food or water, or by not helping them with basic hygiene needs such as bathing or toileting. In another case, a child may be neglected by their parents, who may not provide them with adequate emotional support or fail to enroll them in school.

Neglect can also occur in care homes, where vulnerable individuals may be left without proper care or attention. For example, a resident in a care home may be neglected if they are not provided with enough food or water, or if they are left in bed for long periods of time without any mobility or stimulation.

Neglect can be subtle and hard to detect, and may even be premeditated in some cases. This is why it is important to be vigilant and report any suspicions of neglect to the appropriate authorities, such as social services or regulatory bodies.

Sarah's Story

Sarah was a young woman with autism who had been living in a care home for several years. She was nonverbal, which made it difficult for her to communicate her needs and emotions. However, the staff at the care home were supposed to provide her with the care and support she needed to live a happy and fulfilling life.

Unfortunately, the reality was far from what Sarah deserved. The staff at the care home were neglecting her emotionally and physically, and the neglect was subtle and premeditated. They were more interested in using their phones and socializing with each other than providing Sarah with the care she needed.

The staff often organized events and trips so they could attend to their own errands. For example, they would take Sarah and the other service users on trips to attractive destinations so they could fix their personal caravan. Sarah was sometimes confined to a car all day so that the employee could avoid work and not get caught.

When Sarah's family came to visit, they noticed that she was looking unwell and malnourished. They could see that she was not receiving the care and attention she needed. They asked the staff what was happening, but they were brushed off and told that everything was fine.

Sarah's family became increasingly concerned and decided to take matters into their own hands. They set up a hidden camera in her room, hoping to capture evidence of the neglect. What they saw on the footage was shocking. The staff were often on their phones, ignoring Sarah's needs. She was left alone in her room for hours on end, with no interaction or stimulation.

The family immediately reported their findings to the care home's management and the appropriate authorities. The staff involved were suspended pending an investigation.

The investigation revealed that the staff had been neglecting Sarah and other service users for a long time. They were more interested in their own needs than the needs of the people they were supposed to be caring for. The care home's management were horrified by the findings and made changes to ensure that it never happened again.

Sarah's family eventually moved her to a new care home where she received the care and attention she deserved. However, the emotional and physical scars of her neglect would stay with her for a long time. The neglect that Sarah endured is a stark reminder of the importance of vigilance and accountability in care homes, particularly for those who are nonverbal and unable to speak up for themselves.

Psychological abuse: Psychological abuse is often difficult to detect as it can take many forms, such as bullying, intimidation, or controlling behavior. It can involve making someone feel fearful, anxious, or depressed, or using threats or coercion to manipulate them. Psychological abuse is a form of abuse that can be difficult to detect as it often involves subtle and premeditated actions by the abuser. Staff members in care homes may use a variety of tactics to exert control and manipulate their patients, especially those who are nonverbal and unable to speak up for themselves.

One such tactic is bullying. Staff members may belittle and demean patients, making them feel small and powerless. They may use aggressive body language and facial expressions to intimidate patients, making them feel fearful and anxious. In some cases, they may even use physical force or threats to coerce patients into complying with their demands.

Another tactic is controlling behavior. Staff members may take away patients' personal items or restrict their access to certain areas of the care home, creating a sense of isolation and helplessness. They may also limit patients' communication with family and friends, further isolating them from their support network.

In some cases, staff members may use psychological abuse as a way to manipulate patients for their own benefit. For example, they may withhold food or medication as a way to coerce patients into doing things they don't want to do. They may also use threats or intimidation to keep patients quiet about abuse or neglect that they have witnessed.

Overall, psychological abuse can have a devastating impact on patients' mental and emotional well-being. It can lead to feelings of fear, anxiety, depression, and hopelessness. It can also erode patients' trust in caregivers and make them feel isolated and alone.

It is important for care homes to have policies and procedures in place to prevent psychological abuse and to train staff members on how to recognize and respond to signs of abuse. Patients should also be encouraged to report any instances of abuse or neglect, and care homes should take these reports seriously and take appropriate action to address them. With the right safeguards in place, we can ensure that care homes are safe and nurturing environments for all patients.

In summary, abuse that is difficult to detect can involve emotional, financial, sexual, neglect, or psychological abuse, and can occur in many settings, including care homes, hospitals, and private homes. It is essential to be aware of the signs and symptoms of abuse and report any concerns promptly to the appropriate authorities.

Samanth's Story

Samantha was a young woman with Down syndrome who lived in a care home. She had always been a friendly and sociable person, but over time she became withdrawn and anxious. The staff members at the care home noticed the change in her behavior, but they assumed it was just part of her condition.

However, the reality was far more sinister. Samantha was being subjected to psychological abuse by some of the staff members. They would belittle her and make fun of her in front of other patients, leaving her feeling embarrassed and ashamed. They would also limit her access to her personal items and restrict her movements, making her feel isolated and helpless.

Despite the abuse she was experiencing, Samantha assumed that it was her fault and that she deserved it. She didn't want to complain or speak out, fearing that it would only make things worse. She felt trapped and alone, with nowhere to turn for help.

The staff members responsible for the abuse were premeditated and subtle in their actions. They would often use gaslighting techniques to make Samantha doubt her own perception of reality. For example, they would make comments like "I was just joking, can't you take a joke?" when Samantha became upset or offended by their behavior. They would also make excuses for their actions, saying that they were just trying to help her or that she was being overly sensitive.

The staff members went to great lengths to hide their psychological abuse, knowing that it was difficult to detect and prove. They would make sure that there were no witnesses to their behavior and would often target Samantha when other staff members were not around. They would also use their authority to intimidate her, knowing that she was unlikely to speak out against them.

Eventually, a new staff member at the care home noticed Samantha's withdrawn and anxious behavior and became concerned. They took the time to talk to her and gain her trust, and she eventually confided in them about the abuse she had been experiencing. With the help of the new staff member, Samantha was able to report the abuse and receive the support and care she needed. The staff members responsible for the abuse were held accountable for their actions and were fired from the care home. Samantha received counseling and support to help her heal from the psychological trauma she had experienced.

Samantha's story highlights the importance of recognizing and responding to psychological abuse in care homes. It also underscores the need for greater awareness and training for staff members to ensure that they are providing a safe and nurturing environment for all patients, regardless of their condition. No one should have to experience the kind of psychological abuse that Samantha endured, and it is up to all of us to speak out against it and demand better care for those in need.

DIFFICULTY FOR THE INVESTIGATORS

Investigating allegations of premeditated subtle abuse can be a difficult and complex process, as perpetrators of such abuse are often skilled at concealing their actions and avoiding detection. There are several challenges that investigators may face when trying to gather evidence and build a case against perpetrators of premeditated abuse.

One of the main difficulties is the subtlety and premeditated nature of the abuse itself. Perpetrators may carefully plan and strategize their abusive behavior to achieve their desired outcomes, such as gaining power or control over their victims. They may also be highly skilled at manipulating situations and people to their advantage, often without being detected. This can make it difficult for investigators to identify and document instances of abuse.

Another challenge is the lack of physical evidence. Unlike cases of physical abuse, premeditated abuse may leave little or no physical evidence that can be used in court. Instead, investigators may need to rely on witness statements, surveillance footage, or other forms of circumstantial evidence to build their case.

In addition, victims of premeditated abuse may be hesitant to come forward and report the abuse. They may feel ashamed or embarrassed, or may fear retaliation from their abuser. This can make it difficult for investigators to gather testimony or other forms of evidence that can support the victim's claims.

Finally, perpetrators of premeditated abuse may be skilled at covering their tracks and avoiding detection. They may use tactics such as gaslighting or manipulation to confuse or misdirect investigators, or may destroy evidence that could implicate them in the abuse. This can make it difficult for investigators to gather the evidence needed to prosecute the perpetrator.

If investigators decide that allegations or concerns of abuse are unfounded, it can have several consequences. Firstly, the person who made the allegations or raised the concerns may feel discouraged or dismissed. They may feel that their voice was not heard or that their experience was not taken seriously. This can lead to a breakdown in trust between the individual and the investigators or caregivers, which can make it more difficult for them to come forward in the future.

In addition, the person who was accused of abuse may feel vindicated or may use the decision as a way to continue their abusive behavior. This can put the individual who raised the concerns or made the allegations at further risk of harm, as the perpetrator may feel that they can continue their behavior without consequences.

From a broader perspective, unfounded allegations or concerns can also have negative consequences for the credibility of investigators or caregivers. If there is a perception that allegations are not taken seriously or are dismissed without proper investigation, it can erode trust in the system as a whole. This can make it more difficult for vulnerable individuals to come forward and can create a culture of secrecy and silence around abuse.

To prevent these negative consequences, it is important for investigators and caregivers to take all allegations and concerns seriously, regardless of their perceived merit. They should conduct a thorough and impartial investigation, gathering evidence and interviewing witnesses as needed. If allegations are found to be unfounded, they should be able to provide a clear and transparent explanation for their decision. By treating all allegations and concerns with care and attention, investigators and caregivers can help to create a culture of trust and safety for vulnerable individuals.

Unfortunately, it is not uncommon for social care institutions to cover up abuse, rather than addressing it directly. There are several tactics that may be used to cover up abuse, including moving people to other establishments, using redundancy and scapegoating whistleblowers, and gaslighting those who speak out.

One way that institutions may cover up abuse is by moving people to other establishments. For example, if a resident reports abuse in a care home, the staff may transfer them to another home to prevent them from speaking out further. This tactic can also be used to avoid negative publicity or legal repercussions for the institution.

Another tactic is to use redundancy and scapegoating whistleblowers. This may involve dismissing staff members who have reported abuse, or using them as a scapegoat to deflect attention away from the institution's failings. For example, if a staff member reports abuse in a care home, they may be dismissed for unrelated reasons or blamed for the institution's problems.

Gaslighting is another tactic that may be used to cover up abuse. This involves manipulating individuals into doubting their own perceptions of reality, often through lies or other forms of deception. For example, if a staff member reports abuse, they may be told that they are mistaken or that they are imagining things. This can be a highly effective way to silence whistleblowers and avoid accountability.

Examples of institutions covering up abuse through these tactics are unfortunately all too common. In 2016, the Winterbourne View scandal in the UK exposed widespread abuse of residents with learning disabilities. The institution attempted to cover up the abuse by transferring residents to other homes, dismissing whistleblowers, and using gaslighting to discredit those who spoke out.

Similarly, in the United States, the Penn State University child sex abuse scandal involved the cover-up of abuse by senior staff members, who used tactics such as scapegoating whistleblowers and gaslighting victims to avoid detection and accountability.

Covering up abuse is a serious issue that can have long-lasting and damaging consequences for vulnerable individuals. It is important for institutions to take allegations of abuse seriously and to respond to them with transparency and accountability, rather than attempting to cover them up.

Overall, investigating allegations of premeditated abuse requires careful planning and a thorough understanding of the complexities involved. Investigators must be skilled at gathering evidence, interviewing witnesses, and building a case that can withstand scrutiny in court. By working together to raise awareness of premeditated abuse and to develop effective strategies for investigating and prosecuting perpetrators, we can create a safer and more just society for all.

WARNING: THE DANGER OF INTERNAL INVESTIGATIONS

Internal investigations after whistleblowing can be dangerous for the whistleblower. The internal investigation is typically conducted by the same organization that the whistleblower has reported the concerns about. In some cases, the organization may not take the allegations seriously and may even attempt to cover up the issue.

This can lead to several negative outcomes for the whistleblower. Firstly, the whistleblower may be targeted for retaliation by the organization or by colleagues who are implicated in the misconduct. This can include harassment, intimidation, or even threats of violence.

Secondly, the internal investigation may be biased or incomplete, leading to a lack of accountability for those who are responsible for the misconduct. This can further undermine the credibility of the whistleblower and create a culture of silence within the organization.

Thirdly, the whistleblower may be further traumatized by the investigation process, which can be lengthy, invasive, and emotionally draining. They may be required to provide evidence or testify, which can be a stressful and triggering experience.

In some cases, an internal investigation may even result in the whistleblower losing their job or being ostracized from the organization. This can have a devastating impact on their career, finances, and mental health.

Given these risks, it is important for whistleblowers to seek independent legal and emotional support to protect themselves throughout the investigation process. They should also ensure that they document all of their concerns and report them to the appropriate external regulatory body to ensure that there is transparency and accountability.

THE PSYCHOLOGY OF ORGANIZATIONAL ABUSE

The psychology of organizational abuse refers to the underlying psychological processes and factors that contribute to abuse and neglect within social care organizations. This can include a variety of factors, including power dynamics, organizational culture, and individual attitudes and beliefs.

One key factor that contributes to organizational abuse is power dynamics. In many social care organizations, there is a clear hierarchy of power and authority, with managers and supervisors holding significant power over frontline staff and vulnerable clients. This power imbalance can create an environment in which abusive and neglectful behavior can go unchecked, as employees may be reluctant to speak out against their superiors or may feel powerless to intervene in abusive situations.

Organizational culture is also an important factor in the psychology of organizational abuse. A toxic organizational culture that prioritizes profit over the well-being of clients, or that condones or turns a blind eye to abusive behavior, can contribute to a culture of neglect and abuse.

Individual attitudes and beliefs also play a role in the psychology of organizational abuse. Some employees may hold negative attitudes towards vulnerable populations or may have a callous disregard for their well-being. Others may feel overwhelmed or burnt out by their work, leading to a lack of empathy and caring towards clients.

In order to address the psychology of organizational abuse, it is important to promote a culture of transparency and accountability within social care organizations. This includes providing regular training and support for employees on issues related to abuse and neglect, creating clear policies and procedures for reporting concerns, and implementing systems for monitoring and evaluating the quality of care provided. It also involves challenging toxic organizational cultures and power imbalances and promoting a culture of respect, compassion, and empathy towards vulnerable populations.

There are several reasons why organizational abuse can occur in social care, including:

Power dynamics: Social care organizations often have a clear hierarchy of power and authority, which can create an environment in which abusive and neglectful behavior can go unchecked.

Organizational culture: A toxic organizational

culture that prioritizes profit over the well-being of clients or condones abusive behavior can contribute to a culture of neglect and abuse.

Staffing issues: Understaffing, poor training, and inadequate resources can all contribute to a culture of neglect and abuse, as employees may be overwhelmed or lack the necessary skills and resources to provide adequate care.

Attitudes and beliefs: Negative attitudes towards vulnerable populations, a lack of empathy, and a callous disregard for client well-being can all contribute to abusive and neglectful behavior.

Lack of accountability: In some cases, social care organizations may lack accountability or oversight, which can contribute to a culture of impunity for abusive behavior.

Burnout and stress: High levels of stress and burnout can contribute to a lack of empathy and caring towards clients, which can in turn contribute to abusive and neglectful behavior.

Lack of training and support: Without regular training and support on issues related to abuse and neglect, employees may not know how to recognize or respond to these issues, which can contribute to a culture of neglect and abuse.

It is important for social care organizations to address these underlying factors in order to prevent and address organizational abuse and ensure the well-being of vulnerable clients.

There can be a number of reasons why social care organizations do not always address the concerns that lead to organizational abuse. Some of these reasons include:

Lack of resources: Social care organizations may not have the necessary resources to address the underlying concerns that lead to abuse and neglect, such as inadequate staffing or training.

Lack of awareness: In some cases, organizations may not be aware of the extent of abuse or neglect occurring within their organization, or may not fully understand the underlying factors that contribute to this behavior.

Fear of legal repercussions: Organizations may be hesitant to address abuse and neglect due to concerns about legal liability or negative publicity.

Resistance to change: Addressing the underlying factors that contribute to abuse and neglect may require significant changes to organizational culture or policies, which can be difficult or uncomfortable for some organizations to implement.

Power dynamics: Those in positions of power within social care organizations may be resistant to change or may be more concerned with maintaining their own authority than with addressing concerns about abuse and neglect.

It is important to recognize that addressing concerns about abuse and neglect can be complex and challenging, and may require significant resources and organizational change. However, it is crucial for social care organizations to prioritize the well-being of vulnerable clients and to work towards creating a culture of transparency, accountability, and ethical behavior within the sector.

CLASS PREJUDICE
AGAINST STAFF

Social class prejudice refers to a system of beliefs and attitudes that values individuals or groups based on their social class, often resulting in discrimination or unfair treatment towards those who belong to lower socioeconomic classes. This type of prejudice can manifest in a variety of ways, including negative stereotypes, devaluation of certain professions or types of work, and a lack of access to resources and opportunities.

In the context of social care organizations, social class prejudice can be particularly relevant, as there may be a significant difference in social class between managers and employees. Managers may be more likely to come from higher socioeconomic backgrounds, with greater access to education, resources, and social capital, while employees may be more likely to come from lower socioeconomic backgrounds, with limited access to these resources.

This difference in social class can create a power dynamic that can contribute to social class prejudice and unfair treatment towards employees. For example, managers may be more likely to view their employees as being less educated or less capable, and may make assumptions or decisions based on these beliefs. Employees, on the other hand, may feel undervalued or marginalized, and may be less likely to speak out or advocate for themselves due to fear of retribution.

To address social class prejudice in social care organizations, it is important to promote a culture of respect and inclusivity, and to provide opportunities for all staff to develop their skills and advance in their careers. This can include providing training and mentorship programs, promoting diversity and representation within the organization, and valuing the contributions of all staff, regardless of their social class or educational background.

In addition, it is important to recognize and address the power dynamics that can contribute to social class prejudice, and to work towards creating a more equitable and just workplace for all employees. This may include addressing issues related to pay and benefits, creating opportunities for employee input and participation in decision-making processes, and promoting transparency and accountability in all aspects of the organization.

In many countries, including the UK and the US, social care workers do not require a formal education beyond a high school diploma or equivalent qualification to enter the profession. This means that many social care workers may not have a high level of formal education when they start working in the field.

According to a study conducted by the US Bureau of Labor Statistics, approximately 63% of social care workers in the US have a high school diploma or equivalent qualification, while only 16% have a bachelor's degree or higher. Similarly, in the UK, the majority of social care workers do not have a degree or higher education qualification, although some employers may require or prefer workers to have a relevant diploma or vocational qualification.

While lack of formal education does not necessarily equate to lower skills or competence, it can impact the ability of social care workers to effectively communicate and navigate complex policies and procedures. It can also create barriers for professional development and career advancement within the field.

In recent years, there has been increasing recognition of the importance of education and training for social care workers, particularly in light of the growing complexity and demands of the field. Many employers now require or encourage their workers to pursue relevant training and qualifications, such as diplomas in social care or healthcare-related fields. Some countries have also implemented minimum education requirements for social care workers, such as the requirement for a level 3 qualification in the UK.

While formal education is not always a requirement for entering the social care profession, it is becoming increasingly recognized as an important factor in ensuring high-quality care and promoting professional development and advancement for workers in the field.

Low socioeconomic class and prejudice can influence an individual's perceived credibility when they report safeguarding concerns to a manager from a higher socioeconomic class and education in several ways.

Firstly, individuals from lower socioeconomic classes may be perceived as less educated or less knowledgeable about complex policies and procedures, and therefore may be seen as less credible when reporting safeguarding concerns. This can create a power dynamic in which managers may be more likely to dismiss or discredit the concerns of individuals from lower socioeconomic backgrounds.

Secondly, prejudice towards individuals from lower socioeconomic classes can contribute to negative stereotypes and biases that may influence how managers perceive and respond to safeguarding concerns. For example, a manager may assume that an individual from a lower socioeconomic background is more likely to make false or exaggerated claims, or may be more prone to making mistakes or errors in judgment.

These factors can also be compounded by other forms of prejudice, such as race or ethnicity, which can further erode an individual's perceived credibility and authority when reporting safeguarding concerns. For example, an individual who is both from a lower socioeconomic background and a minority race or ethnicity may face additional barriers and biases that make it more difficult to be taken seriously by managers.

To address these issues, it is important to promote a culture of respect and inclusivity within social care organizations, and to actively work towards challenging stereotypes and biases that can impact the perceived credibility of individuals from lower socioeconomic classes. This can include providing training and support for managers to recognize and address prejudice and bias, as well as promoting diversity and representation within the organization and valuing the contributions of all staff, regardless of their socioeconomic background or educational level. It is also important to provide a safe and supportive environment for individuals to report safeguarding concerns, including protection from retaliation or other forms of negative consequences for speaking out.

Contempt for less educated staff or class prejudice can certainly be included as a reason why social care organizations may not always address the concerns that lead to organizational abuse.

Low educated staff in social care organizations may face significant challenges when making safeguarding disclosures or articulating themselves during cross-examination. These challenges can stem from a variety of factors, including limited literacy skills, difficulty understanding complex legal and policy language, and a lack of confidence in their ability to communicate effectively.

These challenges can have a significant impact on the emotional well-being of staff, who may feel frustrated, powerless, and intimidated by the process of making a safeguarding disclosure or participating in a legal investigation. They may also experience feelings of shame or embarrassment due to their perceived lack of education or language skills, which can further erode their confidence and self-esteem.

To better support low-educated staff in social care organizations, it is important to provide training and resources that are accessible and easy to understand. This can include clear and concise guidelines for making safeguarding disclosures, as well as support and training in effective communication and public speaking.

In addition, staff should be provided with emotional support and counseling throughout the process of making a safeguarding disclosure or participating in a legal investigation. This can include access to mental health services, as well as support groups and peer mentoring programs.

It is also important to recognize the unique contributions and perspectives that low-educated staff bring to social care organizations, and to promote a culture of respect and inclusivity within the workplace. This can include valuing diversity and promoting opportunities for staff to share their experiences and ideas, as well as recognizing and rewarding the contributions of all staff, regardless of their educational background or language skills.

Class Prejudice can manifest in several ways:

1. **Ignoring staff concerns**
2. **Lack of training and support**
3. **Power dynamics**
4. **Lack of representation**

Let's examine these more closely.

Ignoring staff concerns: Staff who are less educated or who come from lower socioeconomic backgrounds may be less likely to be taken seriously by management or may not have access to the same channels of communication or resources as their colleagues. This can make it difficult for them to raise concerns about abuse or neglect within the organization. The issue of ignoring staff concerns is not only limited to staff who are less educated, but also those who come from lower socioeconomic backgrounds. These individuals often face significant barriers to raising concerns about abuse or neglect within their organizations, which can lead to a culture of silence and fear.

One of the primary barriers to raising concerns is a lack of access to the same channels of communication or resources as their colleagues. For example, staff who come from more privileged backgrounds may have access to more training, support, or networking opportunities than those who come from less privileged backgrounds. This can create a perception that their concerns are less important or less credible, which can discourage them from speaking out.

Additionally, staff from lower socioeconomic backgrounds may be less likely to be taken seriously by management, who may view them as less educated or less knowledgeable than their more privileged colleagues. This can create a power dynamic in which staff from lower socioeconomic backgrounds feel that they have no choice but to remain silent, for fear of retribution or being ostracized by their colleagues.

The impact of ignoring staff concerns can be

devastating, both for individual staff members and for the organization as a whole. When concerns about abuse or neglect are ignored, it can lead to a culture of silence and fear, which can contribute to the perpetuation of abuse within the organization. This can have a significant impact on the emotional well-being of staff members, who may feel isolated, unsupported, and powerless.

To address this issue, social care organizations must take a proactive approach to promoting inclusivity and respect for staff from all backgrounds. This can include providing training and support to managers and other decision-makers to recognize and address class prejudice, as well as creating clear channels of communication and resources for staff to report concerns about abuse or neglect.

It is also important to value the contributions of staff from lower socioeconomic backgrounds, and to actively work towards creating a more equitable and just workplace for all staff. This can include providing opportunities for career advancement, professional development, and mentoring for staff from all backgrounds, regardless of their educational background or socioeconomic status. By doing so, social care organizations can create a more inclusive and supportive culture that values the perspectives and contributions of all staff members.

Jame's Story

James had always dreamed of working in social care, ever since he was a young boy growing up in a low-income community. He was passionate about helping others and believed that he could make a difference in the lives of vulnerable people. So when he was offered a job as a care assistant in a local care home, he was thrilled.

At first, James loved his job. He enjoyed working with the residents, helping them with their daily needs, and providing companionship and support. However, after a few months on the job, he began to notice some troubling things happening within the care home.

Some of the residents were being neglected, left in their beds for hours on end without food or water. Others were being verbally abused by some of the other care assistants, who would shout at them or belittle them in front of others. James knew that this was wrong, and he felt that he had a responsibility to speak out.

However, when James raised his concerns with his manager, he was met with a dismissive attitude. His manager told him that he was being overly sensitive and that he should focus on his own work. James was frustrated and felt that his concerns were not being taken seriously.

As time went on, James continued to notice problems within the care home, but he felt increasingly isolated and unsupported. He noticed that some of his colleagues, who came from more privileged backgrounds, seemed to have more access to resources and support than he did. He felt that his concerns were being dismissed because of his socioeconomic background, and he began to doubt his own judgment.

Eventually, James felt that he had no choice but to quit his job. He could no longer stand by and watch as vulnerable residents were neglected and mistreated. It was a difficult decision, as he loved working with the residents and believed that he could make a difference, but he knew that he could not continue to work in an environment where his concerns were ignored.

Looking back on his experience, James realized that he had faced significant barriers to raising his concerns about abuse and neglect within the care home. He felt that his concerns were not taken seriously because of his socioeconomic background and that he did not have the same access to resources and support as his more privileged colleagues. He hoped that one day, social care organizations would do more to promote inclusivity and respect for staff from all backgrounds, so that others would not have to face the same challenges that he did.

Lack of training and support: Staff who are less educated or from lower socioeconomic backgrounds may be less likely to receive the necessary training and support to recognize and respond to abuse or neglect within the organization. In the social care sector, there is a common misconception that only those with higher education degrees or formal qualifications are capable of providing quality care. This often results in prejudice against care workers who do not have a higher education, particularly those who only have a high school education or less.

For example, consider the case of a care worker named Maria. Maria had been working as a caregiver in a residential care home for several years, and although she only had a high school education, she was passionate about providing the best possible care for the residents. One day, Maria noticed that one of the residents was becoming increasingly withdrawn and unresponsive. She tried to engage the resident in conversation, but the resident wouldn't respond. Maria became concerned and decided to raise her concerns with her manager.

However, when Maria brought up her concerns with her manager, she was dismissed and told that she didn't have the necessary education or training to make a proper judgment about the resident's condition. Maria was upset and frustrated, feeling like her concerns were not being taken seriously because of her educational background.

This type of prejudice is not only unfair but can also have serious consequences for vulnerable people in care. Care workers who do not have a higher education or formal qualification are often the ones who spend the most time with residents and are most familiar with their behaviors and needs. Dismissing their concerns simply because they do not have a higher education can lead to serious issues being overlooked and potentially cause harm to those in care.

It is important for social care organizations to recognize the valuable contributions that care workers with different educational backgrounds can make. By providing adequate training and support, organizations can ensure that all staff members, regardless of their educational background, are equipped to provide the best possible care for residents. Additionally, social care organizations should value and respect the concerns of all staff members and create a culture of open communication and collaboration, where all staff members feel heard and valued.

Power dynamics: Staff who are less educated or from lower socioeconomic backgrounds may be more vulnerable to abuse or exploitation within the organization, particularly if they are in lower-level positions and have less power or authority. In the social care sector, power dynamics can play a significant role in creating an environment where staff who are less educated or from lower socioeconomic backgrounds are more vulnerable to abuse or exploitation. This is especially true for those in lower-level positions who may have less power or authority than their colleagues.

For example, imagine a care home where a care assistant named Tom has been working for several years. Tom comes from a lower socioeconomic background and has only completed high school. Despite his lack of formal education, Tom is passionate about providing quality care to the residents and is well-liked by both residents and colleagues.

However, one day Tom notices that one of his colleagues, a higher-level staff member, is mistreating a resident. Tom is unsure of what to do as he is worried that speaking out could put his job at risk. He knows that the higher-level staff member has more authority and power within the organization, and he fears that his concerns will not be taken seriously.

This kind of power dynamic can create a culture of fear and silence within an organization, where staff members who are less educated or from lower socioeconomic backgrounds feel vulnerable and unsure of how to raise concerns. This can be compounded by the fear of losing their job or being retaliated against by colleagues or management.

It is important for social care organizations to recognize these power dynamics and work to create an environment where all staff members feel empowered to raise concerns and have their voices heard. This can be achieved through training and education on abuse and exploitation in the workplace, as well as creating clear policies and procedures for reporting concerns. Additionally, organizations should create a culture of support and advocacy for all staff members, regardless of their background or position within the organization. By addressing power dynamics and creating a safe and supportive environment, social care organizations can help ensure the safety and well-being of both staff members and those in their care.

Lack of representation: Staff who are less educated or from lower socioeconomic backgrounds may be underrepresented in leadership positions or decision-making roles within the organization, which can contribute to a culture of neglect or abuse. In the social care sector, staff who are less educated or from lower socioeconomic backgrounds may also face challenges due to a lack of representation in leadership positions or decision-making roles within the organization. This can have significant consequences for both the organization and the individuals in their care.

For example, imagine a care home where the management team is made up of individuals who all have advanced degrees and come from affluent backgrounds. They may have a limited understanding of the challenges faced by staff members who are less educated or from lower socioeconomic backgrounds, which can result in policies and practices that are not inclusive or sensitive to the needs of all staff members.

This lack of representation can also contribute to a culture of neglect or abuse, as those in leadership positions may not fully appreciate the impact of their decisions on staff members and those in their care. This can lead to a situation where concerns raised by staff members from lower socioeconomic backgrounds are not given the attention they deserve, and issues of neglect or abuse go unaddressed.

To address this issue, social care organizations must prioritize diversity and inclusion in their hiring and promotion practices. They must actively work to recruit and retain staff members from diverse backgrounds, and create opportunities for staff members to advance into leadership positions. Additionally, they should seek out the input and perspectives of all staff members, regardless of their background, to ensure that policies and practices are inclusive and reflective of the needs of all stakeholders.

By addressing the lack of representation among staff members from lower socioeconomic backgrounds, social care organizations can create a more inclusive and supportive culture that prioritizes the safety and well-being of all staff members and those in their care.

Addressing class prejudice and ensuring that all staff are treated with respect and dignity is crucial for preventing organizational abuse and promoting a culture of ethical behavior within social care organizations. This can include providing equal access to training and support, ensuring that all staff have a voice and are taken seriously when raising concerns, and promoting diversity and representation within the organization.

THE VALUES OF AN ABUSIVE EMPLOYEE AND ORGANISATION

It is relatively easy to find information on good social care values and legislation that guide the work of social care professionals. Social care professionals are expected to uphold these values and follow the legislation while providing services to individuals. Therefore, there is no need to cover them extensively in this book. We will do that later.

However, it is equally important to examine and address any values that may be in opposition to positive social care values. Some employees may hold values that are in opposition to the positive social care values, such as prejudice or discrimination. These values can lead to abusive or neglectful behavior towards individuals receiving social care services. By examining these values, employees can work towards aligning them with positive social care values, which can ultimately lead to improved outcomes for the individuals receiving social care services.

Moreover, understanding the dark side of human nature is also crucial in social care.

It is important for social care professionals to understand that anyone, regardless of their position or background, can exhibit abusive or neglectful behavior towards vulnerable individuals. By acknowledging this reality, social care professionals can be more vigilant and aware of any signs of abuse or neglect, and work towards preventing them.

By promoting a culture of continuous learning and personal development, social care organizations can create an environment where employees are encouraged to examine their own values and beliefs and to work towards aligning them with positive social care values. This can ultimately lead to improved outcomes for the individuals receiving social care services and a safer and more positive work environment for the employees.

Organisations and employees who engage in abuse or neglect often try to justify their behavior by espousing certain values or beliefs. These may include:

Efficiency and productivity: In some cases, employees or organisations may prioritise efficiency and productivity over the well-being of service users. This can result in neglect or abuse, as employees may feel pressured to cut corners or take shortcuts in order to meet performance targets.

Cost-saving measures: Similarly, organisations

may implement cost-saving measures that result in inadequate resources or understaffing. This can lead to neglect or abuse, as employees may not have the time or resources to provide proper care.

Hierarchy and authority: In some cases, employees may feel that they are justified in mistreating service users because of their position of authority. This can be particularly prevalent in situations where there is a significant power differential between the employee and service user.

Stigma and prejudice: Negative attitudes towards certain groups of service users can contribute to neglect or abuse. For example, employees may hold stigmatising beliefs about people with mental health issues or disabilities, which can lead to neglect or mistreatment.

Lack of training and education: Employees who have not received adequate training or education may lack the knowledge or skills necessary to provide proper care. This can lead to unintentional neglect or abuse, as employees may not understand the impact of their actions on service users.

It is important to note that these values and beliefs are not inherently negative, and may be expressed in a variety of contexts. However, when they are used to justify neglect or abuse, they can have serious consequences for service users.

To prevent abuse and neglect, it is important for organisations and employees to recognise the impact of their values and beliefs on their behaviour. This can involve addressing implicit biases, providing adequate training and resources, and prioritising the well-being of service users above all else.

THE VALUES OF THE ABUSER IN SOCIAL CARE

Values are deeply ingrained beliefs or principles that guide an individual's behaviour and decision-making. In social care, values play a crucial role in how employees interact with service users and the quality of care they provide. However, when an individual's values are conditioned or arbitrary, they can lead to abuse or neglect of service users.

Conditioned values are beliefs that an individual has acquired over time through socialisation and cultural norms. These values are often taken for granted and may be deeply ingrained in an individual's psyche, to the point where they are not consciously aware of them. In social care, conditioned values can contribute to a culture of neglect or abuse. For example, an employee who has grown up in a culture that values toughness and stoicism may be less likely to respond to a service user's emotional needs, leading to neglect.

Arbitrary values, on the other hand, are beliefs that are not based on any objective or rational criteria. They may be influenced by personal biases or prejudices and can lead to discriminatory or abusive behaviour towards service users. For example, an employee who holds arbitrary values that certain service users are less deserving of care or attention may neglect their needs.

Both conditioned and arbitrary values can be dangerous in social care, as they can lead to abuse or neglect of service users. To prevent this, organisations should provide employees with training and education on cultural competence and diversity, as well as regularly monitor employee behaviour to identify any potential biases or values that may be contributing to abuse or neglect. Additionally, it is important for organisations to create a culture of accountability and transparency, where employees are encouraged to speak up about any concerns they may have regarding the treatment of service users. Conditioned and arbitrary values that are in opposition to social care values can lead to abusive or neglectful behaviour towards service users.

Some examples of these values include:

1. Paternalism
2. Stigma
3. Authoritarianism
4. Individualism
5. Consumerism
6. Control
7. Punishment
8. Tokenism
9. Blame
10. Compliance

Let's examine these more closely.

Paternalism: An employee who holds conditioned values that service users are less knowledgeable and less capable of making decisions about their own care may disregard their wishes or fail to involve them in decision-making. Paternalism is a phenomenon where an employee assumes an authoritative or paternalistic role in their interactions with service users. This may occur when an employee holds conditioned values that service users are less knowledgeable and less capable of making decisions about their own care, resulting in the employee disregarding their wishes or failing to involve them in decision-making.

Paternalism can have a significant impact on service users, as it can lead to feelings of disempowerment and disengagement from their own care. This can result in a lack of motivation to engage with the care provided and a decline in overall wellbeing.

The belief that service users are not capable of making decisions about their own care may be rooted in the employee's personal upbringing or cultural background. For instance, an employee may have been raised in a culture where elders are expected to be cared for by their children and are not given the autonomy to make decisions about their own care. This conditioning may influence their approach to caring for service users and result in paternalistic behaviours.

It is important for employees to recognize and address their own paternalistic tendencies in order to provide person-centered care that respects the autonomy and choices of service users. This can be achieved through training and education that promotes values of respect, dignity, and empowerment.

In addition, organizations should create a culture that encourages open communication and transparency, where service users are involved in decision-making about their care. This can help to break down the paternalistic attitudes of employees and promote a more person-centered approach to care.

By examining the negative values and biases that can be held by employees, social care organizations can help their staff to understand the dark side of human nature and how it can manifest in their work. This can help employees to develop a deeper sense of empathy and respect for service users, and ultimately provide better care.

The Story of Emma's experience of Paternalism

Emma had always been a fiercely independent woman, even as she grew older and her health began to decline. But when her mobility started to decrease, her family decided that it was time for her to move into a care home to receive the support she needed.

Emma was initially hesitant, but her family assured her that the care home was one of the best in the area, with a reputation for providing excellent care. Emma reluctantly agreed, but from the moment she arrived, she felt like she had lost all control over her life.

The care home staff seemed to treat her like a child, constantly telling her what to do and where to go, and ignoring her requests to make decisions about her own care. Emma found it difficult to express her concerns, as the staff were dismissive of her opinions, telling her that they knew what was best for her.

Emma's frustration with the staff's attitude continued to grow, but she didn't know what to do. She felt like she was trapped, with no way to voice her concerns or take control of her own life again.

One day, Emma's family came to visit and noticed that she seemed unhappy and withdrawn. When they asked her what was wrong, Emma finally opened up about how the staff treated her.

Her family were shocked and immediately reported the situation to the care home management. It became clear that the staff had been operating under a paternalistic mindset, believing that they knew what was best for Emma, rather than involving her in her own care.

The care home management took action to address the issue, providing staff training on the importance of respecting service users' autonomy and involving them in their own care decisions. Emma's family also advocated for her, ensuring that her voice was heard and that her needs were being met.

Although it took some time, Emma eventually regained control over her own life and was able to live in the care home with dignity and respect. Her experience highlighted the importance of treating all service users with respect and involving them in their own care decisions, rather than assuming that the care provider always knows best.

Stigma: An employee who holds conditioned values that service users with mental health conditions are dangerous or unpredictable may stigmatize them, leading to a lack of empathy or understanding and potentially discriminatory or abusive behaviour. Stigma towards service users with mental health conditions is a serious issue that can lead to discrimination and abusive behavior. Employees who hold conditioned values that service users with mental health conditions are dangerous or unpredictable may stigmatize them, leading to a lack of empathy or understanding. This can result in service users being denied equal opportunities and access to services, being isolated or excluded, and being subjected to physical or psychological abuse.

The effects of stigma can be profound, and can contribute to feelings of shame, fear, and worthlessness among service users. This, in turn, can lead to a deterioration of their mental health and well-being, as well as a lack of trust in the care system.

Employees who hold stigmatizing beliefs about service users with mental health conditions may also be more likely to engage in discriminatory behavior, such as denying access to services or treatment, withholding medication, or using physical or chemical restraints unnecessarily. This type of behavior not only violates the human rights of service users, but also undermines the principles of social care and the importance of treating all service users with dignity and respect.

It is crucial that employees are educated on the harmful effects of stigma and the importance of treating all service users equally, regardless of their mental health condition. This can be achieved through training programs, policies and procedures, and by creating a culture of respect and understanding within the workplace. By promoting empathy, compassion, and inclusivity, employees can help to break down the barriers of stigma and provide high-quality care to all service users.

STORY OF SAMANTHA
AND THE STIGMA:

Samantha had been living in a residential care home for individuals with mental health conditions for several years. During that time, she had developed a close relationship with one of the care workers, named Sarah. However, Samantha started to notice a change in Sarah's behaviour towards her.

Sarah became more distant and would avoid interacting with Samantha as much as possible. When Samantha asked what was wrong, Sarah told her that she was becoming too difficult to handle and was taking up too much of her time. Samantha was confused and hurt by this, as she had always thought she and Sarah had a good relationship.

Things got worse when Samantha began to notice that other care workers were treating her differently too. They would talk down to her, ignore her requests for help, and sometimes even avoid going into her room altogether. Samantha couldn't understand why she was suddenly being treated this way.

One day, Samantha overheard two care workers talking about her. They were saying that Samantha was "one of those crazy ones" and that they didn't want to deal with her anymore. Samantha realized that they were stigmatizing her because of her mental health condition, and that Sarah had likely started to see her in the same way.

Samantha felt alone and isolated in the care home. She no longer felt like she could trust the people who were supposed to be caring for her. She tried to speak to the care home manager about what was happening, but felt like she was not being taken seriously. Samantha knew that she needed to find a way to get help before the situation got worse.

Eventually, Samantha was able to contact an advocacy group for people with mental health conditions. They helped her to make a formal complaint about the way she was being treated. After an investigation, it was discovered that several care workers, including Sarah, had been stigmatizing Samantha and treating her differently because of her mental health condition. The care home took action and provided training for all staff members to address the stigma and discrimination faced by people with mental health conditions. Samantha was moved to a different unit within the care home, and the care workers who had mistreated her were disciplined.

While Samantha was glad that action had been taken to address the abuse, she couldn't help but feel the scars of the experience. She felt betrayed by Sarah, who had been a friend to her. Samantha knew that stigma and discrimination were common in society, but she never expected to face it from those who were meant to be caring for her.

Authoritarianism: An employee who holds arbitrary values that their role as a care worker grants them total authority over service users may act in ways that undermine the dignity and autonomy of service users. Authoritarianism is an arbitrary value that some care workers may hold, leading to a dangerous power dynamic between the service user and the caregiver. This may manifest in a range of behaviours, such as disregarding service users' wishes and treating them as subordinates rather than equal partners in their own care.

In an authoritarian culture, care workers may believe that they have complete control over service users and can make decisions for them, without involving them in the decision-making process. This can lead to a lack of respect for the service user's autonomy and dignity. For example, a care worker may refuse to allow a service user to make choices about their own care, or may belittle their suggestions and ideas.

Such arbitrary beliefs can contribute to a culture of abuse, as the caregiver may feel entitled to use their power and control over service users. The result is a loss of dignity and autonomy for the service user, who may be subjected to restrictive or harmful practices.

To combat authoritarianism, it is essential that care workers are educated about the importance of respecting the autonomy and dignity of service users. They must be trained to understand that service users have the right to make choices about their own care and be involved in the decision-making process.

Furthermore, it is crucial that care organizations promote an environment of collaboration and partnership between service users and care workers. Service users should be treated with the utmost respect and dignity, with their opinions and preferences valued and incorporated into their care plans. Only then can we truly combat authoritarianism and create a safe and empowering environment for service users in social care settings.

The Story of Oliver and the Authoritarian

Oliver was a 25-year-old man with Down syndrome who required support with daily living tasks. He had a bubbly personality and loved spending time with his family and friends. He lived in a residential care home where he received 24-hour support from care workers.

One of the care workers, Sarah, had a tendency to be overly authoritative with the residents. She believed that her role as a care worker gave her complete authority over the residents and that they should comply with her every demand. This led to her mistreating Oliver on several occasions.

Oliver loved playing basketball, and he often played with other residents in the courtyard. However, Sarah believed that Oliver should not be playing basketball as she considered it a dangerous activity for someone with Down syndrome. She ordered Oliver to stop playing and sit in his room instead. When Oliver protested, Sarah grabbed him by the arm and dragged him back to his room. On another occasion, Oliver wanted to wear his favorite t-shirt to a family gathering. However, Sarah believed that the t-shirt was not appropriate and forced him to wear something else. When Oliver refused, Sarah physically restrained him and forced him to change.

Oliver's family noticed a change in his behavior and asked him if everything was okay. Oliver confided in them about the mistreatment he had been receiving from Sarah. They immediately reported the incidents to the care home manager.

The care home manager investigated the allegations and found that Sarah had been mistreating Oliver and other residents. Sarah was disciplined and eventually fired from the care home. The care home also implemented additional training for all staff members on the importance of respecting the autonomy and dignity of residents.

Oliver's family were relieved that the abuse had been addressed and that Oliver was receiving the care and support he deserved. They were grateful that Oliver had the courage to speak out and report the mistreatment he had been experiencing.

Individualism: An employee who holds arbitrary values that personal achievement and ambition are more important than collective welfare may neglect the needs of service users in favour of their own career advancement or interests. Individualism in social care can also manifest in an employee altering a care plan to their own opinion of how they think the service should be delivered to a certain client. This can happen when an employee disregards the needs and preferences of the service user and imposes their own ideas of what is best for the service user.

Such employees may fail to recognize that each service user is an individual with unique needs and preferences, and that the care plan should be tailored to meet their specific needs. Instead, they may impose their own ideas and opinions, leading to inadequate or inappropriate care.

This type of individualism can be especially harmful in cases where the service user has a disability or is unable to communicate their needs clearly. The employee may assume that they know what is best for the service user, leading to neglect or abuse.

To prevent this type of individualism in social care, it is important for employees to receive training on person-centered care, where the service user is at the center of the care plan and their needs and preferences are taken into consideration. Additionally, employees should be encouraged to listen to service users and their families, and to work collaboratively with other staff members to develop care plans that meet the unique needs of each service user.

Overall, individualism in social care can lead to neglect or abuse of service users and undermines the core values of social care. It is essential for employees to understand the importance of collective welfare, collaboration, and putting the needs of service users first to ensure that the values of social care are upheld.

Johns Encounter with Individualism

John, a young man with developmental disabilities, was excited to move into his new residential home where he could live independently with support from the care staff. However, he soon found himself feeling isolated and neglected by the care staff.

One staff member, named Sarah, was particularly individualistic in her approach to care. She often talked about her personal goals and ambitions rather than focusing on the needs and desires of the service users. Sarah would often cut corners to finish her work faster and move onto her own personal interests, leaving John without the support he needed.

An example of Sarah's individualistic approach in social care occurred when she promised John a day trip to a nearby park. However, on the day of the outing, Sarah did not have any plans to take John out and instead confined him to the car for the entire day while she played games on her phone. John was left feeling disappointed and neglected, and his needs and wishes were ignored in favour of Sarah's personal interests.

John asked Sarah if he could go on a day trip to a nearby museum, but she dismissed his request, saying that it was not part of his care plan and it was not in her schedule. John felt disappointed and unheard, but he didn't know how to speak up for himself.

Another time, John became ill and asked for Sarah's help. However, she refused, saying that she was too busy and that he should take care of himself. John felt helpless and alone, but he didn't know how to speak up for himself.

As time went on, John began to feel more and more neglected by the care staff. He started to lose weight, and his mental health began to suffer. One day, a visiting family member noticed John's deteriorating condition and raised concerns with the management.

It was discovered that Sarah had been neglecting her responsibilities as a care staff and focusing solely on her own interests. She was fired, and the management implemented more training and support for the remaining staff to prevent such individualistic behaviour from happening again.

In this scenario, Sarah's individualistic values prioritized her own comfort and entertainment over John's needs and well-being. Her lack of empathy and compassion for John led to inadequate and harmful care. Additionally, her behaviour undermined the core values of social care, such as putting the needs of service users first, collaboration, and teamwork.

To prevent individualistic values from influencing social care, it is essential that employees receive training on the importance of collective welfare, empathy, and compassion. Furthermore, the importance of putting the needs of service users first should be emphasized, and employees should be encouraged to work together with colleagues, service users and their families to provide quality care. This way, employees can better understand the impact of their actions on service users, and the values of social care can be upheld.

Consumerism: An employee who holds arbitrary values that service users are customers rather than individuals in need of care may prioritize profit or efficiency over the well-being of service users. Consumerism is a value system that places a high value on the acquisition of material goods and services. In the context of social care, an employee who holds arbitrary consumerist values may view service users as customers rather than individuals in need of care. This individualistic mindset may lead to the prioritization of profit or efficiency over the well-being of service users.

Such an employee may approach their work with a business mindset, viewing service users as a means to achieve financial gain. They may prioritize the financial success of the organization over the quality of care provided to service users, which can lead to neglect or abuse. For example, a care worker may prioritize meeting financial targets over providing adequate care for service users, leading to short-staffing or cutting corners to save costs.

The focus on profit may also lead to a culture of competition between employees, where staff are motivated by financial incentives rather than the well-being of service users. This can lead to a lack of collaboration and teamwork, with staff competing with each other for financial rewards or recognition rather than working together to provide quality care.

Moreover, consumerist values may lead to the commodification of service users, where their individual needs and desires are ignored in favour of efficiency and profitability. For example, a care worker may prioritize completing tasks quickly over engaging in meaningful interactions with service users or taking the time to understand their individual needs.

To prevent consumerist values from influencing social care, it is important for organizations to prioritize the well-being of service users over financial gain. Care workers should be trained to view service users as individuals with unique needs and desires, rather than customers to be serviced efficiently. Furthermore, staff should be incentivized and recognized for providing high-quality care, rather than financial gain or productivity. This way, the values of social care can be upheld, and service users can receive the care and support they deserve.

Sophie Becomes a Commodity

Sophie, a service user with a learning disability, was excited when her social worker told her that she would be moving to a new residential home. Sophie had been living in a crowded and understaffed home, and she hoped that the new home would provide her with better care and support.

When she arrived at the new home, she was pleasantly surprised by the clean and spacious facilities. However, her excitement soon turned to disappointment when she realized that the care staff treated her more like a customer than a person with unique needs and desires.

Sophie's care plan was focused solely on meeting her basic needs, such as food, shelter, and hygiene, rather than addressing her individual preferences and interests. The care staff often rushed through their tasks and paid little attention to Sophie's emotional well-being or social needs.

Sophie's biggest disappointment came when she was not allowed to participate in activities that interested her. She loved to paint and draw, but the care staff would not allow her to attend art classes because they were not covered by her care plan. Instead, she was offered a range of activities that did not interest her, such as bingo and group exercise.

Sophie felt frustrated and powerless. She felt like she was just a source of profit for the home, and that her individual needs and preferences were not important. She became withdrawn and depressed, and her mental health began to suffer.

It was only when Sophie's family members intervened and spoke with the management of the home that changes were made. The management recognized the importance of addressing the unique needs and desires of each service user and implemented changes to ensure that each service user received individualized care and support.

Sophie's care plan was revised to include her interest in art, and she was given access to art classes. The care staff were also trained to focus on the individual needs and preferences of service users, rather than treating them like customers.

Sophie's mental health improved, and she started to feel like her voice was being heard. She felt like she was more than just a source of profit for the home and that her individual needs and preferences were being valued.

In this scenario, Sophie suffered due to the care home's value of consumerism, which prioritized profit and efficiency over the well-being and individual needs of service users. The care staff treated Sophie like a customer rather than a person with unique needs and desires, leading to inadequate and harmful care. It was only when the management recognized the importance of individualized care and support that Sophie's needs were properly addressed.

Control: An employee who holds conditioned values that individuals with challenging behaviour are willful or disobedient may use restrictive measures such as restraints or seclusion to control their behaviour, rather than seeking to understand and address the underlying reasons for the behaviour.Control is a conditioned value that an employee may hold in social care that involves exerting power over service users to regulate their behaviour. An employee who holds arbitrary values that individuals with challenging behaviour are willful or disobedient may use restrictive measures such as restraints or seclusion to control their behaviour, rather than seeking to understand and address the underlying reasons for the behaviour.

This behaviour may stem from a lack of understanding or training on positive behaviour support principles, which prioritize understanding the root cause of behaviour and addressing it in a way that is respectful and least restrictive. Instead, an employee who holds the value of control may believe that the use of physical or psychological restraint is an acceptable solution to behaviour that is deemed challenging or difficult.

Such behaviour can lead to a culture of abuse within the organisation, where the needs and dignity of service users are disregarded, and they are treated as objects to be controlled rather than individuals with autonomy and agency. The use of restraints or seclusion without proper training or justification can result in physical or psychological harm to the service user and contribute to feelings of powerlessness, frustration, and mistrust.

Moreover, the use of control-based measures can exacerbate challenging behaviour, leading to a cycle of reactive responses that fail to address the underlying issues. This can be harmful to the service user and create a difficult working environment for staff members who are not trained in positive behaviour support or do not hold the value of control.

To prevent the value of control from influencing social care, it is essential that employees receive training on positive behaviour support principles and the importance of understanding and addressing the underlying causes of behaviour. Furthermore, the use of restraints or seclusion should only be used as a last resort, with clear guidelines and justification. This way, the dignity and autonomy of service users can be respected, and the values of social care can be upheld.

The Story of Sarah and Control

Sarah had been living in a residential care home for adults with developmental disabilities for several years. She had been diagnosed with autism and had difficulty communicating her needs and wants. Despite these challenges, she was able to establish a good relationship with most of the care staff.

One day, a new staff member, named James, joined the care team. James had a very authoritarian approach to care and believed that the service users needed to be controlled and disciplined. He often used physical restraints and other aversive interventions to manage their behaviour.

Sarah's behaviour had become challenging, and James was determined to "fix" her. He believed that Sarah needed to learn to follow rules and obey authority, and he was not afraid to use force to achieve this. Whenever Sarah exhibited behaviour that James deemed inappropriate, he would use restraints to control her, or put her in seclusion.

As a result, Sarah became increasingly withdrawn and fearful of the care staff. She felt like she had lost her sense of agency and control over her own life. She no longer felt like she could trust the staff to respect her boundaries and needs.

Sarah's family noticed a change in her behaviour

and raised concerns with the care home management. An investigation revealed that James had been using excessive force and had violated Sarah's rights. He was dismissed from his job, and the management implemented more training and support for the remaining staff to prevent such behaviour from happening again.

Despite the corrective action taken by the management, the damage had already been done. Sarah was left with physical and emotional scars from the abuse she experienced. Her trust in the care staff had been shattered, and she had to undergo additional therapy to help her cope with the trauma.

This situation illustrates how an authoritarian approach to care can have detrimental effects on service users. It also highlights the importance of upholding the values of social care, such as dignity, respect, and the right to self-determination. The well-being of service users should always be the top priority, and care staff should be trained to use positive reinforcement and proactive strategies to manage behaviour, rather than relying on punishment and control.

Punishment: An employee who holds conditioned values that individuals with challenging behaviour should be punished for their actions may use aversive interventions such as physical restraints or verbal reprimands, rather than positive reinforcement or other proactive strategies to promote positive behaviour. Punishment is a value system that emphasizes retribution and consequences over compassion and understanding. In social care, an employee who holds conditioned values of punishment may perceive individuals with challenging behaviour as deserving of punishment for their actions, rather than trying to understand and address the underlying causes of the behaviour.

Such employees may use aversive interventions such as physical restraints or verbal reprimands, as a means of punishing individuals with challenging behaviour. This approach can lead to a deterioration in the individual's well-being, self-esteem, and trust in the care system. The use of punishment in social care can be detrimental to the core values of dignity, respect, and empathy that underpin social care practice.

Moreover, punishment as a value system may be more prevalent in care systems that prioritize compliance and control over positive behaviour support. Employees who hold such values may see punishment as a quick and easy solution to managing challenging behaviour, rather than taking the time to develop individualized, proactive support plans that address the root causes of the behaviour.

To prevent punishment as a value system from influencing social care, employees should be trained in positive behaviour support and encouraged to prioritize compassion and understanding in their work. Positive reinforcement, proactive strategies, and individualized support plans should be emphasized over aversive interventions, which can have harmful and long-lasting effects on the well-being of service users. A shift in values towards a more positive and proactive approach to supporting individuals with challenging behaviour can help to promote their well-being, dignity, and autonomy, and ensure that the core values of social care are upheld.

Maggie's Punishment

Maggie was a 40-year-old woman with a history of mental health issues. She had been admitted to a mental health care facility after experiencing a severe episode of depression. Maggie was placed in a specialized unit where she would receive treatment for her condition.

Maggie's assigned care worker, Mark, had a punitive approach towards mental health care. Mark believed that individuals with mental health conditions needed to be disciplined and punished for their behaviour. Whenever Maggie displayed any signs of disruptive behaviour, Mark would reprimand her harshly and use aversive interventions like restraints to control her behaviour.

Maggie found it difficult to cope with Mark's approach to care. She felt that her needs and wishes were being ignored, and that Mark was only interested in punishing her for her behaviour. Maggie's condition worsened under Mark's care, and she became increasingly isolated and withdrawn.

One day, Maggie's condition deteriorated significantly, and she experienced a severe episode of self-harm. Mark responded by restraining her in a prone position for an extended period, which caused Maggie to suffer physical and emotional harm. Maggie was left traumatized by the experience, and her mental health suffered further as a result.

The management of the care facility investigated the incident and discovered that Mark's approach to care was not aligned with the values of social care. They provided training and support to Mark to help him understand the importance of positive reinforcement and other proactive strategies to promote positive behaviour, rather than punitive measures like restraints.

Maggie was eventually transferred to a different unit with care workers who had a more compassionate and understanding approach to mental health care. With the right support and care, Maggie was able to recover from her condition and regain her independence.

This experience highlights the dangers of a punitive approach to care in social care. Employees who hold the value of punishment may use aversive interventions that can cause harm to service users. To prevent this from happening, employees should receive training on the importance of positive behaviour support and the use of non-aversive interventions in social care. The well-being and dignity of service users should always be the top priority in social care, and punitive measures should only be used as a last resort in exceptional circumstances.

Tokenism: An employee who holds arbitrary values that individuals with challenging behaviour can be placated by receiving rewards or incentives may rely on token systems that offer only superficial or temporary rewards, rather than addressing the individual's underlying needs and preferences. Tokenism is an arbitrary value system that places emphasis on superficial or symbolic gestures to address complex issues, rather than implementing meaningful change. In social care, an employee who holds tokenistic values may focus on offering superficial or temporary rewards to individuals with challenging behaviour rather than addressing their underlying needs and preferences.

For example, an employee may implement a token system where service users receive rewards for exhibiting positive behaviour. However, if the rewards offered are not meaningful or do not align with the individual's needs and preferences, they may not be effective in promoting long-term positive behaviour. Additionally, token systems that only offer superficial or temporary rewards may contribute to a lack of engagement and motivation for service users.

Furthermore, an employee who relies on tokenistic values may also fail to address the underlying issues that contribute to challenging behaviour. For instance, an individual may exhibit challenging behaviour due to an unmet need, such as a need for increased social interaction or sensory stimulation. In such a case, a token system that only focuses on rewards and incentives will not address the underlying need and may perpetuate the challenging behaviour.

Tokenism in social care undermines the core values of person-centred care and may further marginalize individuals with challenging behaviour. It is crucial that employees receive training on the importance of meaningful engagement, addressing underlying needs, and implementing individualized approaches to promote positive behaviour.

In conclusion, tokenistic values in social care may lead to a lack of engagement, superficial rewards, and a failure to address underlying needs, further perpetuating challenging behaviour. Therefore, it is essential that social care employees recognize the limitations of token systems and prioritize person-centred approaches that address the underlying needs and preferences of service users.

The Story of Julie and the Tokens

Julie was a 45-year-old woman with intellectual disabilities who had been living in a group home for several years. The staff in the home were responsible for Julie's daily care, including managing her finances and supporting her with daily living activities.

One day, Julie's support worker, Rachel, came up with a new idea to improve Julie's motivation and engagement in daily activities. Rachel suggested that they start using a token system where Julie would earn tokens for completing certain tasks or goals, which she could then exchange for rewards such as sweets or extra TV time.

At first, Julie was excited about the token system and eagerly participated in the tasks assigned to her by Rachel. However, as time went on, Julie became increasingly disillusioned with the system. She felt like her accomplishments were only being recognized if she earned tokens, rather than being valued for their own sake. She also felt like the rewards offered were trivial and didn't really make a difference in her life.

As Julie became more disengaged with the token system, Rachel became more insistent that Julie participate. She would withhold rewards if Julie didn't earn enough tokens, and would often scold her for not trying hard enough. Julie began to feel like her efforts were never enough, and that she was being punished for not conforming to the token system.

The token system had become a form of tokenism, where Julie's individual needs and preferences were being ignored in favour of a superficial reward system. Julie's support worker, Rachel, had become so focused on the token system that she had forgotten to consider Julie's unique needs and preferences.

Eventually, Julie's family noticed that she was becoming increasingly withdrawn and unhappy, and they raised concerns with the management of the group home. After investigating, the management recognized that the token system was not working for Julie and was causing her distress. They stopped the use of the token system and implemented a more person-centred approach to Julie's care.

Through person-centred care, Julie's needs and preferences were taken into account, and her support was tailored to her individual needs. She was no longer being forced to participate in a token system that did not work for her, and instead, she was able to engage in activities that brought her joy and satisfaction. The values of social care, such as person-centred care and individual needs, were upheld, and Julie was finally able to receive the care and support she deserved.

Blame: An employee who holds arbitrary values that individuals with challenging behaviour are solely responsible for their behaviour may blame them or their caregivers for the behaviour, rather than taking a collaborative and compassionate approach to behaviour support. Blame is an arbitrary value system in which an employee perceives individuals with challenging behavior as solely responsible for their actions. This arbitrary value can negatively impact the quality of care provided to these individuals. When an employee subscribes to this value system, they may be inclined to blame individuals or their caregivers for the behavior rather than adopting a collaborative and compassionate approach to behavior support.

This approach is not only counterproductive but may also lead to further challenges for the individual. Instead of identifying and addressing the underlying cause of the behavior, an employee who subscribes to this value system may focus solely on the behavior and the consequences of the behavior.

This approach may lead to a punitive and confrontational approach to addressing challenging behavior, leading to the further escalation of the behavior. It also ignores the importance of positive behavior support strategies, such as proactive intervention plans that address the underlying causes of the behavior.

Furthermore, this approach may create a culture of blame and finger-pointing, which can create a hostile work environment and undermine the quality of care provided to individuals with challenging behavior. It may also foster a culture of fear, in which caregivers may be hesitant to report challenging behavior for fear of being blamed or criticized.

To prevent blame from influencing social care, it is essential that employees receive training on collaborative and compassionate approaches to behavior support. The importance of identifying and addressing the underlying causes of the behavior should be emphasized, and employees should be encouraged to adopt positive behavior support strategies.

By addressing challenging behavior in a compassionate and collaborative manner, employees can create a culture of support and understanding that promotes the welfare of individuals with challenging behavior. This approach can improve the quality of care provided to individuals with challenging behavior and promote a more positive work environment for caregivers.

The Story of Maria and Blame

A client named Maria was receiving social care services due to her physical disabilities. She was unable to move around without the help of a wheelchair and relied on the care staff to support her with daily activities. One day, Maria was struggling to communicate her needs to a care staff member named John, who was particularly prone to blaming the service users for their difficulties.

John held the arbitrary value that individuals with disabilities are responsible for their own care and should be able to communicate their needs clearly. He had little patience for those who struggled to express themselves, and he often became frustrated with Maria when she had difficulty communicating.

One day, Maria was unable to communicate her needs, and John became frustrated and blamed her for not trying hard enough. He even suggested that her disability was an excuse for her lack of effort. This left Maria feeling frustrated, helpless and isolated.

As a result of John's blameful attitude, Maria began to feel more anxious and worried about her ability to communicate her needs to the care staff. She began to lose trust in the care staff, feeling like they were not able to support her fully. This caused her mental health to suffer, and she became increasingly withdrawn and isolated.

It was only when another care staff member noticed Maria's deteriorating condition that the issue was raised with the management. They were shocked to hear about John's behaviour, and they took immediate action to address the issue. John received training on the importance of empathy and compassion in social care, and he was encouraged to approach care with a more collaborative and supportive attitude.

Maria finally received the care and support she deserved, and her mental health improved significantly. However, the damage had already been done, and Maria was left with lasting emotional scars as a result of John's blameful attitude. The incident served as a reminder of the importance of empathy, compassion, and understanding in social care, and the need to avoid blameful attitudes towards vulnerable service users.

Compliance: An employee who holds arbitrary values that individuals with challenging behaviour should comply with social norms or expectations may focus on conformity and obedience, rather than supporting the individual's unique needs and preferences. Compliance is a personal value system that emphasizes adherence to social norms and expectations. In social care, an employee who holds arbitrary compliance values may prioritize conformity and obedience over the individual needs and preferences of service users, particularly those with challenging behaviours.

This can manifest in various ways, such as an employee imposing strict routines or expectations on service users without considering their individual preferences or needs. For example, an employee may insist that a service user participate in a certain activity or therapy, even if it causes distress or is not enjoyable for the individual. This approach can be particularly damaging for individuals with challenging behaviours, as it can lead to further frustration, anxiety and challenging behaviour.

Moreover, an employee who prioritizes compliance may fail to recognize the importance of individuality and uniqueness in social care. They may focus solely on social norms and expectations, disregarding the individual needs and preferences of service users. This can result in care plans that are not tailored to the unique needs and strengths of the individual, leading to ineffective or even harmful care.

Additionally, an employee who prioritizes compliance may be resistant to new or innovative approaches to care, particularly those that challenge existing norms or expectations. They may be reluctant to consider alternative approaches to behaviour support, even if they have been shown to be more effective or person-centred. This resistance to change can be particularly detrimental to the quality of care provided to service users.

To prevent compliance values from influencing social care, it is essential that employees receive training on the importance of individuality, uniqueness and person-centred care. The values of collaboration, empathy, and compassion should also be emphasized, and employees should be encouraged to work together with colleagues, service users and their families to provide quality care that is tailored to the unique needs and preferences of each individual. This way, employees can better understand the impact of their actions on service users, and the values of social care can be upheld.

The Story of Jenny and Compliance

Jenny had been living in a social care facility for several months. She had a mild intellectual disability and needed support for activities of daily living. The care staff provided her with assistance for her meals, personal care, and activities. However, Jenny often felt that her voice was not heard by the staff, and that she had no control over her own life.

One day, the care staff introduced a new policy requiring all service users to adhere to a strict schedule for meals, activities, and bedtime. Jenny struggled with the new routine, as she preferred to eat at different times and engage in activities of her own choosing. When she voiced her concerns, the care staff dismissed her, stating that she needed to comply with the new policy.

Jenny felt frustrated and ignored by the care staff. She felt that her unique needs and preferences were not being respected. As a result, she became more withdrawn and disengaged from the social activities and interactions with the staff.

Despite her protests, Jenny was forced to comply with the strict schedule, which led to her feeling more anxious and distressed. She felt like her life was not her own, and that she had no control over her own decisions.

The care staff's emphasis on compliance and strict adherence to policy undermined Jenny's autonomy and dignity. Instead of working collaboratively with Jenny to find a routine that worked for her, they imposed a one-size-fits-all approach. This approach left Jenny feeling powerless and unable to exercise any control over her own life.

To prevent such experiences, social care organizations should prioritize the empowerment and autonomy of service users. Policies and routines should be developed collaboratively with service users and should be flexible to accommodate their unique needs and preferences. Moreover, care staff should receive training on the importance of respecting service users' autonomy and dignity, and the value of person-centered care.

THE DARK TETRAD

The concept of the dark tetrad was proposed by psychology researchers Delroy Paulhus and Kevin Williams in 2002. It is an extension of the dark triad, which includes three personality traits: narcissism, Machiavellianism, and psychopathy. The dark tetrad adds a fourth trait, sadism, to the mix.

The dark tetrad is based on the idea that certain personality traits are linked to a propensity for malevolent behavior. These traits have been studied extensively in the field of personality psychology, and research has shown that they can be measured using self-report questionnaires.

The scientific background of the dark tetrad lies in the study of personality and its influence on behavior. Personality is a complex construct that encompasses a variety of traits, beliefs, and behaviors. Researchers have identified a number of personality traits that are associated with negative outcomes, including aggression, criminal behavior, and unethical conduct.

The dark tetrad is an attempt to identify the specific personality traits that are most closely associated with malevolent behavior. It is based on empirical research and has been studied extensively in the field of personality psychology.

While some researchers have criticized the dark tetrad for being too narrow in its focus, others have praised it for shedding light on the complex interplay between personality and behavior.

The Dark Triad is a personality construct consisting of three traits: narcissism, Machiavellianism, and psychopathy. More recently, the Dark Tetrad has been proposed, which includes the aforementioned traits plus sadism. Together, they form what is known as the "dark diad" or "dark tetrad".

These traits are characterized by a lack of empathy and concern for others, a willingness to manipulate and exploit others for personal gain, and a tendency to engage in impulsive and aggressive behavior. These traits can explain abusive behavior in social care because they involve a disregard for the well-being of others and a desire for power and control.

Individuals who possess these traits may be drawn to careers in social care as they offer opportunities to exert power and control over vulnerable individuals. Additionally, the hierarchical nature of many social care organizations may provide an environment in which these individuals can exercise their desire for dominance over others.

Abusive behavior in social care may manifest as neglect, emotional abuse, physical abuse, or sexual abuse. The individual may engage in manipulative tactics to gain control over the individual or may exploit their vulnerabilities for personal gain.

It is important to note that not all individuals who exhibit traits of the dark diad will engage in abusive behavior, and not all abusive behavior is a result of these traits. However, understanding the potential for these traits to contribute to abusive behavior can help to identify and address abusive behavior in social care. Training and education on recognizing and addressing abusive behavior can help to prevent the abuse of vulnerable individuals in social care settings.

The Dark Tetrad is a set of four personality traits that are associated with negative and harmful behavior towards others. The four traits are:

1. **Narcissism:**
2. **Machiavellianism:**
3. **Psychopathy:**
4. **Sadism:**

Let's examine these more closely.

NARCISSISM:

a personality trait characterized by a grandiose sense of self-importance, a lack of empathy for others, and a need for admiration. Narcissism is a personality trait that can significantly impact the behaviour of social care employees and ultimately affect the well-being of the clients they serve and the staff they work with. A social care employee with narcissistic traits can display a grandiose sense of self-importance, believing that their needs and desires are more important than those of others. This may lead them to prioritize their own goals and ambitions over the needs of clients, resulting in neglect or even harm.

A lack of empathy for others is another characteristic of narcissism, meaning that a social care employee with this trait may struggle to understand or connect with the experiences and emotions of clients and their families. They may fail to recognize the emotional and psychological impact of illness, disability, or abuse on clients, leading to inadequate care and support.

The need for admiration is also a key aspect of narcissism, meaning that social care employees with this trait may seek constant praise and attention from others. This can lead to a focus on superficial or performative acts rather than providing genuine care and support to clients.

Additionally, social care employees with narcissistic traits may exhibit controlling behaviour, seeking to dominate and manipulate clients and staff to maintain their perceived sense of power and control. This can result in a toxic work environment, causing stress and harm to clients and colleagues alike.

Overall, narcissism can pose a significant risk to the well-being of clients and staff in social care. It is important for social care organizations to recognize and address these traits in their employees through training and support, as well as implementing measures to promote a culture of empathy, collaboration, and client-centered care.

Story of the Narcissist
Care Professional

One client, named Jane, had recently moved into a new residential home to receive support with her daily activities due to her physical disability. She was assigned a care worker named Mark, who was known for his grandiose sense of self-importance and lack of empathy towards others. Despite Jane's attempts to communicate her needs and preferences, Mark would often dismiss her requests and impose his own ideas and schedule on her care plan.

For instance, Jane had requested to have her meals at a certain time and in a specific way, but Mark would often disregard her wishes and instead serve her food whenever he pleased, or serve her meals that she didn't particularly like. When Jane expressed her dissatisfaction, Mark would belittle her and make her feel like she was being unreasonable.

Additionally, Mark would often talk about his own achievements and accomplishments, making Jane feel unheard and unimportant. He would also criticize her in front of other staff members and service users, causing her to feel embarrassed and humiliated.

One of Jane's colleagues, named Maria, had also experienced Mark's narcissistic behavior. Maria had raised concerns about Mark's approach to care, but he had dismissed her concerns and instead turned the situation around to make it seem like she was incompetent and incapable of performing her own duties.

Mark's behavior not only impacted Jane's well-being but also created a toxic work environment for his colleagues. His lack of empathy and disregard for others' needs and feelings put both clients and staff members at risk.

Eventually, Jane and Maria raised their concerns to the management of the residential home, and Mark was dismissed from his position. The management also provided training and support for the remaining staff to prevent such behavior from happening again.

Asocial care workers with narcissistic personality traits can be detrimental to the well-being of clients and colleagues. Their lack of empathy and inflated sense of self-importance can lead to neglect, abuse, and a toxic work environment. It is crucial that social care workers receive training and support to recognize and address such behavior to ensure the safety and well-being of those they are meant to care for.

MACHIAVELLIANISM:

a personality trait characterized by a manipulative and exploitative approach to others, a lack of moral principles, and a willingness to use deceit and manipulation to achieve personal goals. A social care employee who exhibits Machiavellianism as a personality trait can pose significant risks to the well-being of both clients and colleagues. Such individuals are often motivated by personal gain and will manipulate and exploit others to achieve their goals, often at the expense of others.

In the context of social care, a Machiavellian employee may manipulate clients to achieve their own ends, such as gaining control over the client or advancing their own career. For instance, they may deceive clients into following their own agenda rather than supporting the clients' interests or wishes. Such an approach may lead to clients feeling exploited or manipulated, eroding the trust and rapport between the client and care worker.

In addition, a Machiavellian employee may also manipulate colleagues to achieve their goals, which can lead to a toxic work environment. For example, they may spread false information or engage in smear campaigns against colleagues to gain a competitive edge or promote their own career. Such behavior can erode trust and collaboration within the workplace, leading to a breakdown in team dynamics and jeopardizing the quality of care provided to clients.

Furthermore, a Machiavellian employee may not have a moral compass, which can lead to unethical behavior, including fraud and abuse. They may engage in unethical conduct, such as falsifying documentation, to achieve their goals or to cover up their misdeeds. This can lead to significant harm to clients and staff alike, as well as the reputation of the organization.

In conclusion, the Machiavellian trait can pose a significant risk to the well-being of clients and colleagues in social care. It is essential that employees are screened for this trait during recruitment and that ongoing training and support are provided to prevent such behavior. Additionally, organizations must develop a culture that promotes ethical behavior, collaboration, and accountability to prevent the negative impact of Machiavellianism on social care.

The Story of the Macavellian Care Worker

Sarah was a care worker in a residential home for individuals with intellectual disabilities. She had a charming and confident demeanor that seemed to impress the management team during her interview, but her co-workers and the service users noticed that there was something off about her.

One of Sarah's colleagues, Mary, noticed that Sarah was always trying to undermine her authority and take credit for her work. Mary suspected that Sarah was trying to make herself look good to the management team at her expense. Sarah was always finding ways to blame Mary for things that were not her fault, and Mary found herself constantly on edge and feeling like she was walking on eggshells around Sarah.

One of the service users in the home, Alex, noticed that Sarah was always making promises to him that she never kept. For example, Sarah promised Alex that they would go on a day trip to the beach, but when the day arrived, she claimed that she had never promised anything and that Alex was mistaken. Alex felt frustrated and hurt, as he had been looking forward to the day trip for weeks.

Sarah's manipulative and exploitative behavior only got worse over time. She would often gossip and spread rumors about her colleagues, causing a toxic work environment. She also showed favoritism towards certain service users, giving them preferential treatment over others.

It was only after multiple complaints from both her colleagues and the service users that the management team started to investigate Sarah's behavior. They found evidence that she had been manipulating and exploiting both her colleagues and the service users for her own personal gain.

Sarah was eventually terminated from her job, but the damage had already been done. Mary and Alex were left feeling violated and hurt by Sarah's Machiavellian behavior. It took some time for them to trust other care workers again, but eventually, with the help of supportive colleagues and a supportive community, they were able to move on from the experience.

PSYCHOPATHY:

a personality trait characterized by a lack of empathy or remorse for others, a disregard for social norms, and a tendency towards impulsive and antisocial behavior. A social care employee with psychopathic traits could pose a significant risk to the well-being of clients and colleagues. Psychopathy is characterized by a lack of empathy, which can make it difficult for the individual to understand and respond to the needs of others. This lack of empathy can lead to a disregard for the safety and well-being of clients and colleagues, and a tendency to prioritize their own desires and needs over those of others.

Individuals with psychopathic traits may also display a disregard for social norms, including laws and ethical standards. They may engage in impulsive and reckless behavior that can put themselves and others at risk, such as using physical force or engaging in sexual misconduct. They may also be willing to manipulate and exploit others for personal gain, including financial gain or to advance their career.

Psychopathic individuals may have a superficial charm that allows them to manipulate others into trusting them, making it difficult for colleagues or clients to recognize their true nature. They may also engage in behavior that is aggressive or threatening, which can create a hostile work environment for colleagues or a frightening environment for clients.

In social care, the risks associated with psychopathic traits are particularly concerning because of the vulnerable nature of the clients being served. Individuals with psychopathic traits may see vulnerable clients as easy targets for exploitation or abuse, and may be more likely to engage in behavior that is harmful or neglectful towards them.

To prevent individuals with psychopathic traits from posing a risk in social care, it is essential that employers conduct thorough background checks and psychological assessments before hiring new staff. Additionally, training should be provided on ethical standards and appropriate boundaries, as well as on recognizing and responding to abusive or manipulative behavior. Clients and colleagues should also be encouraged to report any concerning behavior or incidents to management, and management should have procedures in place to investigate and address such reports.

Story of The Psychopath

Sophie was a client in a social care home for adults with intellectual disabilities. She was non-verbal and required assistance with all activities of daily living. Sophie's main caregiver was a staff member named James, who had been working in the home for several years. Initially, James appeared to be friendly and caring towards Sophie, and she seemed to respond well to him. However, over time, James' behaviour towards Sophie began to change. He became increasingly dismissive of her needs and would often ignore her when she tried to communicate with him. He would also isolate Sophie from the other residents and staff, taking her to a separate room where he would spend long periods of time alone with her.

Sophie's colleague, a fellow care worker named Maria, noticed James' behaviour and became concerned. She tried to speak to James about the way he was treating Sophie, but he brushed off her concerns and became defensive.

As time went on, Sophie's behaviour started to change. She became withdrawn and anxious, and would often cry when James was around. She also began to display signs of physical abuse, including bruises and scratches on her arms and legs.

Maria became increasingly alarmed by Sophie's condition and decided to report James to the management.

One of James' other colleagues also made a report that he had overheard James bragging about manipulating a service user into giving him money. The colleague became suspicious and reported the incident to the management team. The management team investigated the incident and found evidence that James had been coercing and manipulating the service user into giving him money for several months.

During the investigation, other concerning behavior was discovered, including James isolating service users from their families and friends, and prioritizing his own personal interests over the needs of the service users. Additionally, the management team discovered that James had falsified records and lied about completing tasks, such as administering medication to the service users.

Further investigation revealed that James exhibited traits of psychopathy, such as a lack of empathy, remorse, and a disregard for social norms. It became clear that James' actions were not only harmful to the service users but also put his colleagues and the reputation of the care home at risk.

The management team terminated James' employment and reported his behavior to the appropriate authorities. The service users impacted by James' actions were provided with additional support and counseling to help them cope with the trauma they experienced. The care home also implemented additional training and screening processes to prevent future incidents of this nature.

In this case, James' psychopathic tendencies were discovered through a combination of whistleblowing by a colleague, investigation by the management team, and the identification of patterns of concerning behavior. The care home's response highlights the importance of having clear policies and procedures in place for identifying and addressing concerning behavior in care workers, as well as providing support for service users and colleagues impacted by such behavior.

SADISM:

a personality trait characterized by a pleasure in inflicting pain or humiliation on others, whether physically or emotionally. A social care employee with a sadistic personality trait would pose a significant risk to the well-being of clients and colleagues. This personality trait is characterized by a pleasure in inflicting pain or humiliation on others, whether physically or emotionally. Such an employee may derive satisfaction from seeing others suffer or may enjoy asserting their power and control over others.

In social care settings, an employee with sadistic tendencies may use physical or emotional abuse to exert their dominance over clients and colleagues. They may intentionally cause harm to others through actions such as neglect, verbal abuse, or physical violence. This can result in physical and emotional trauma for clients, leading to long-term mental health issues and a breakdown of trust in care providers.

Moreover, an employee with sadistic tendencies may also target their colleagues, bullying or harassing them to assert their dominance and control. This can create a toxic work environment, leading to high levels of stress, low morale, and burnout among employees.

It is crucial to identify employees with sadistic tendencies during the recruitment process and provide ongoing training and support to prevent them from causing harm to clients and colleagues. Additionally, protocols for reporting and investigating instances of abuse must be put in place to ensure that employees with sadistic tendencies are held accountable for their actions.

An employee with a sadistic personality trait poses a severe risk to the well-being of clients and colleagues in social care settings. It is crucial to identify and address such employees to uphold the core values of social care and ensure the safety and well-being of those in need of care and support.

The Story of the Sadist Social Care Worker

Samantha had been living in a residential care home for adults with developmental disabilities for three years. She had been doing well under the care of the staff, until a new member joined the team, named David. David was often described as cold, distant and unapproachable by the other staff members, but no one thought much of it until Samantha's behaviour began to change.

At first, Samantha became withdrawn and uncommunicative, which was very unlike her bubbly and talkative personality. Her roommate, Lisa, also noticed a change in her behaviour. She became more anxious and agitated, and started having nightmares. Lisa had always been close to Samantha, so she decided to ask her what was wrong. At first, Samantha was reluctant to talk, but eventually she confided in Lisa that David had been acting inappropriately towards her.

Samantha explained that David would often come into her room and make inappropriate comments about her appearance. He would touch her in a way that made her feel uncomfortable, and he would often smirk or laugh when she protested. Samantha was too scared to report David's behavior to the other staff members, fearing that he would retaliate against her.

Lisa was horrified by what she had heard and knew she needed to do something. She immediately reported the abuse to the care home manager, who took the matter seriously and began an investigation. It was soon discovered that David had a history of sadistic behavior towards vulnerable adults, and he was immediately suspended pending a full investigation.

Further investigation revealed that David had been engaging in sadistic behavior towards several other clients as well. He had been using his position of power to inflict pain and humiliation on the clients, often under the guise of "training" or "discipline". David had been using physical restraints and verbal abuse to control the clients, often laughing or smirking when they expressed their distress.

David was subsequently dismissed from his job

and his actions were reported to the authorities. The care home management team implemented more rigorous training and screening procedures for new staff members to prevent similar incidents from happening in the future.

Samantha and the other clients affected by David's sadistic behavior were provided with counseling and support to help them recover from the trauma they had experienced. Although the care home was able to take steps to prevent future abuse, the harm caused by David's sadistic tendencies had a long-lasting impact on the clients' well-being and trust in their care providers.

These four traits are often referred to as the "Dark Tetrad" because they are associated with a range of negative behaviors and outcomes, including aggression, violence, bullying, and harassment.

In the context of social care, these traits can manifest in various ways. For example, a care worker who is high in narcissism may prioritize their own needs and desires over the needs of the service users, leading to neglect or abuse. A care worker who is high in Machiavellianism may manipulate and exploit service users or colleagues for personal gain. A care worker who is high in psychopathy may engage in impulsive and antisocial behavior that puts service users at risk. A care worker who is high in sadism may take pleasure in inflicting pain or humiliation on service users.

By understanding the traits of the Dark Tetrad, we can identify individuals who may be at risk of engaging in abusive or harmful behavior towards others in the social care setting. This knowledge can inform training and development programs for care workers, as well as inform hiring and screening processes to ensure that individuals with these traits are not employed in social care.

CONCLUSION

The book provides a detailed and insightful look into the dark realities of abuse within the adult social care system. Through the exploration of historical and current cases, the book exposes the pervasive nature of abuse despite the existence of legislation designed to protect vulnerable individuals.

The accounts of Winterbourne View and Whalton Hall serve as powerful reminders of the devastating consequences that can occur when abusive behavior goes unchecked. Additionally, the book delves into the challenges faced by whistleblowers, who often suffer significant professional and personal consequences for speaking out against abuse.

One of the most valuable aspects of the book is its examination of the various techniques used to suppress whistleblowers, including intimidation, harassment, and dismissal. The book also highlights the difficulties faced by investigators in identifying and investigating subtle forms of abuse, such as emotional and psychological abuse.

Another important topic discussed in the book is the issue of class prejudice against staff within the social care system. The book notes that staff members from lower socio-economic backgrounds are often subjected to prejudice and stereotyping, which can contribute to a toxic work environment and increase the risk of abusive behavior.

The book also provides an in-depth exploration of the values and traits commonly exhibited by abusive employees, including narcissism, Machiavellianism, and psychopathy, as well as the terrifying traits described in the dark triad.

Ignoring the insights and recommendations of Subtle Abuse could have dangerous consequences for vulnerable individuals in the adult social care system. The book highlights the persistent presence of abuse, even with existing regulations and protections, and underscores the need for ongoing efforts to prevent and address abusive behavior. Failure to take this issue seriously could result in continued harm and trauma for those in care, as well as perpetuate a toxic and abusive work environment for social care staff.

It is worth noting that Subtle Abuse stands out as a rare example of a social care book that addresses the darker side of human nature. Many books in the field of social care focus on positive outcomes and successes, and may shy away from discussing the realities of abuse and neglect. This could be due to a variety of reasons, such as a desire to maintain a positive image of the social care system, a lack of awareness or acknowledgement of the problem, or fear of backlash or negative consequences for whistleblowers.

The issue of abuse in the social care system can also be challenging to address and investigate, particularly in cases of emotional or psychological abuse. The complexity and subtlety of these forms of abuse can make them difficult to recognize and prove, and may require specialized training and expertise. Additionally, the stigma and shame associated with abuse can make it difficult for individuals to come forward and report instances of abuse, further complicating efforts to prevent and address it.

Despite these challenges, it is essential to address the darker side of human nature in the social care system. Subtle Abuse serves as a valuable resource for those seeking to better understand and combat abuse in the adult social care system. By shedding light on the motivations and behaviors that underpin abuse, the book offers insights and recommendations for creating a safer and more supportive environment for vulnerable individuals and social care staff alike.

The dark subjects covered in Subtle Abuse are essential for social care workers and organizations as they provide crucial insights into the realities of abuse and neglect within the system. By confronting these difficult topics head-on, social care workers can gain a deeper understanding of the complexities and challenges involved in preventing and addressing abusive behavior. This understanding can help to inform policy and practice, ultimately leading to a safer and more supportive environment for vulnerable individuals.

Furthermore, by acknowledging the darker side of human nature, social care organizations can begin to break down the stigma and shame associated with abuse. This can help to create a culture of openness and accountability, where instances of abuse are taken seriously and addressed promptly. In this way, confronting the dark subjects covered in Subtle Abuse can lead to positive change and improvements in the social care system.

However, it is important to acknowledge that many people may loathe the content of this book due to its disturbing and unsettling subject matter. The stories and examples presented in the book are often difficult to read and may trigger strong emotions in readers. Additionally, some may be reluctant to confront the realities of abuse within the social care system, either due to fear, denial, or a desire to maintain a positive image of the system.

Despite these challenges, it is essential that social care workers and organizations confront the darker aspects of their work. By doing so, they can better protect vulnerable individuals, hold abusive individuals accountable, and create a safer and more supportive environment for all. While the content of Subtle Abuse may be difficult to stomach, its insights and recommendations are vital for improving the social care system and ensuring the safety and dignity of all individuals within it.

The principle that the only way to find something evil is to know and study its nature is based on the idea that understanding the nature of evil is essential to prevent or counteract it. Just as ancient humans would study the behavior of predators in order to protect themselves and their loved ones, modern society must study the nature of evil to protect vulnerable individuals and prevent harm.

In the context of social care, studying the nature of abuse and neglect is crucial to identifying and preventing abusive behavior. By understanding the traits and behaviors commonly exhibited by abusive individuals, social care workers and organizations can better recognize warning signs and take action to prevent harm. This knowledge can also inform policy and practice, leading to the implementation of stronger protections for vulnerable individuals and increased accountability for abusive behavior. However, studying the nature of evil can also be challenging and unsettling, as it may require confronting difficult and disturbing subject matter. This can be particularly difficult in the context of social care, where the goal is to promote the health and well-being of vulnerable individuals. However, it is essential to acknowledge that abuse and neglect exist within the social care system and to take proactive steps to prevent and address it.

The principle of studying the nature of evil also highlights the importance of ongoing learning and professional development for social care workers. As new research and insights emerge, social care workers must remain informed and up-to-date on best practices for preventing and addressing abuse and neglect. This ongoing learning can help to ensure that social care workers are equipped with the knowledge and skills needed to protect vulnerable individuals and create a safer and more supportive environment for all.

The principle that the only way to find something evil is to know and study its nature is essential to preventing and addressing abusive behavior within the social care system. By understanding the nature of abuse and neglect, social care workers and organizations can better protect vulnerable individuals and promote a safer and more supportive environment for all.

I hope this book serves as a powerful and sobering reminder of the ongoing challenges faced in the fight against abuse within the adult social care system. It offers valuable insights and recommendations for addressing these challenges, including increased training and support for staff, stronger protections for whistleblowers, and greater transparency and accountability in investigations of abuse. Anyone working in the social care field or concerned about the welfare of vulnerable individuals will find this book to be an important and thought-provoking read.

If you found this book useful please let me know. I am a bit of a Narcissist and need the praise.

Thanks Muchly

Alexander Hylton Parker

arccstic@gmail.com

www.ingramcontent.com/pod-product-compliance
Lightning Source LLC
Chambersburg PA
CBHW070326220526
45467CB00001B/53